Imaging Trauma and Polytrauma in Pediatric Patients

Vittorio Miele • Margherita Trinci
Editors

Imaging Trauma and Polytrauma in Pediatric Patients

Springer

Editors
Vittorio Miele
Department of Emergency Radiology
S. Camillo Hospital
Rome
Italy

Margherita Trinci
Department of Emergency Radiology
S. Camillo Hospital
Rome
Italy

ISBN 978-3-319-08523-4 ISBN 978-3-319-08524-1 (eBook)
DOI 10.1007/978-3-319-08524-1
Springer Cham Heidelberg New York Dordrecht London

Library of Congress Control Number: 2014951705

Printed on acid-free paper

Springer is part of Springer Science+Business Media (www.springer.com)

To Giacomo and Chiara, Vittorio and Carlo

Foreword

Over the past two decades, there has been a change in the conception of emergency and trauma radiology. The increasing awareness that appropriate and rapid therapeutic action in life-threatening situations result from the skillful interpretation of emergency radiologists in dedicated radiology facilities has led to the identification of emergency radiology as distinct specialty of diagnostic imaging.

Cross-sectional imaging with computed tomography (CT), ultrasound (US) and magnetic resonance imaging (MRI) plays a pivotal role in the evaluation of trauma patients, especially in the pediatric population in which particular attention is to be given to the patient's triage, indication to imaging, scanning protocols and radiation dose exposure. Actually, if there is no doubt that high energy traumas and deceleration injuries demand an accurate multi-organ evaluation with CT imaging, in everyday pratice most children come to our observation with bruises and "low energy traumas" following sports activity at school or at home. In these cases, the first diagnostic approach is not (and cannot be!) CT, but X-rays and US whose diagnostic accuracy is highly improved thanks to the use of contrast agents (CEUS).

This book comes from the deep knowledge and extensive experience acquired on a daily basis by a group of dedicated radiologists, highly attentive to all aspects of trauma radiology in the pediatric population. Thus, the book covers from patient's management to the technical aspects of each single modality in their appropriate clinical context, passing through US and MRI of musculoskeletal injuries, child abuse and medico-legal issues.

However, the attention of Dr. Vittorio Miele and the dedication of Dr. Margherita Trinci to this text go beyond the purposes of a simple "how-to" handbook. Particularly, I personally know Vittorio's care and contribution to the growth of emergency radiology during the past 25 years and his daily commitment to set up a team of dedicated and motivated colleagues who share with him enthusiasm and passion for acutely-ill patients. This is, in my personal opinion, the additional value of this book which does not only give practical advices on the use and interpretation of imaging but tries to give a "tailored approach", a "vision" of a delicate and controversial issue, which is often overemphasized, despite trauma being the commonest cause of sudden death and a major cause of disability in children.

I am confident that this book will become an integral part of the core curriculum for residents and fellows but will be also very much in demand in postgraduate training and daily practise for radiologists involved in the emergency radiology setting.

Castel Volturno, Italy Mariano Scaglione

Contents

Pediatric Polytrauma Management

1

Vittorio Miele, Ilenia Di Giampietro, Stefano Giannecchini, Caterina Pizzi, and Margherita Trinci

1.1 Introduction

Trauma is the cause of over 45 % of deaths in children aged 1–14 years; more than 5,000 traumatic deaths occur in this age group every year, 80 % of which are unintentional and 47 % are directly related to road accidents [1, 2]. The mortality estimates of children admitted to hospital following an accident are uniformly low; however, most trauma deaths occur at the scene and then prior to the arrival at a health facility. This is the reason why the overall mortality rates have been underestimated.

Statistics show that the mortality rate, as a result of road accident, has risen dramatically among children in the age group of 13 years and above, since a young car occupant is much more vulnerable. On the other hand, pedestrian and bicycle crashes predominate in the age group of 5–9 years. Drowning is the cause of about 10–15 % of injuries, burns account for about 5–10 %, and falls account for 2 % of deaths [3–5]. Furthermore, the percentage of children suffering abuses should not be underestimated, and in fact, even though a significant reduction in these events has occurred, about 13 % of deaths in the age group of 1–14 is related to homicide [2, 6] (Table 1.1).

In children, the area more frequently affected by trauma is the skull [7, 8], then the associated thoracic–abdominal injuries [1–3, 7, 8]. Since multiple injuries are common among children, the emergency physician has to assess all the organs of an injured child, independent of the real mechanism of the trauma.

Even if the principles of polytrauma management are identical both in children and in adults, the optimal pediatric patient care requires a specific understanding

V. Miele (✉) • I. Di Giampietro • S. Giannecchini • C. Pizzi • M. Trinci
Cardiovascular and Emergency Radiology Department, S. Camillo Hospital,
C.ne Gianicolense, 87, Rome 00152, Italy
e-mail: vmiele@sirm.org; Ilenia.digiampietro@gmail.com; giannecchinis@gmail.com;
caterpizzi@gmail.com; margherita.trinci@libero.it

V. Miele, M. Trinci (eds.), *Imaging Trauma and Polytrauma in Pediatric Patients*,
DOI 10.1007/978-3-319-08524-1_1

Table 1.1 Leading causes of traumatic deaths in children 1–14 years of age in the United States 2004 [2, 6]

Etiology	%
Motor vehicle accidents	38.2
Homicide	13.3
Drowning	13.2
Burn	9.1
Suicide	5.4
Suffocation	4.5
Other	16.3

Table 1.2 Anatomic differences in adults and children and implications for pediatric trauma management

The child's body size allows for a greater distribution of traumatic injuries; therefore, multiple trauma is common
The child's greater relative body surface area also causes greater heat loss
The child's internal organs are more susceptible to injury based on more anterior placement of the liver and spleen and less protective musculature and subcutaneous tissue mass
The child's kidney is less well protected and more mobile, making it very susceptible to deceleration injury
The pancreas is less protected by the abdominal muscles and fat and is therefore more susceptible to injury from impact against the spine
The child's head-to-body ratio is greater, the brain less myelinated, and cranial bones thinner, resulting in more serious head injury

of some important anatomical, physiological, and psychological differences that play a significant role in the assessment and management of a pediatric patient [9]. A comprehensive outline of the anatomical differences and of their implications in a polytrauma patient is listed in Table 1.2.

In general, the body of a child has higher elasticity, so that even severe internal injuries may occur without any recognizable external signs. Children are particularly at risk of severe injuries since, proportionally to weight–height ratio, they have bigger and more adjacent solid organs, less subcutaneous fat, and less muscular protection than adults.

Besides, in relation to the adverse ratio head–body and the larger body surface in relation to weight, each force will be more widely distributed making the most significant probability that multiple lesions may occur. The imbalance between the large body surface and the weight leads the child to a greater amount of heat loss in relation to a higher evaporation.

All these factors prove that the energy level and the caloric requirement of a polytrauma child are much larger than that of an adult. Physiologically, each child responds to the trauma in a different way depending on the age and severity of the injury, but each procedure relative to free water and electrolyte maintenance is to be amplified.

Unlike adults, children have a great ability to maintain their blood pressure despite a significant and acute blood loss (from 25 to 30 %). Small changes in heart rate, arterial pressure, and perfusion of the extremities may indicate an imminent presentation of cardiorespiratory failure and, therefore, should not be neglected. Finally, children do not have the ability to better manage an environment that is not their usual, and, for this reason, they are excessively irritable, making their health status assessment even more difficult.

Recent data have shown that 25 % of children involved in road accidents will show signs of post-traumatic stress disorder following the discharge [10]. The pediatric patient needs a calm, sometimes unconventional, approach in such a way as to reduce their state of anxiety.

1.2 Primary Survey

The primary objective of management of a young trauma patient is to identify and address immediate life-threatening injuries.

The initial assessment and the arrangement of possible resuscitation procedures can and should be rapid (5–10 min); it is convenient to follow the logical sequence A–B–C–D–E (airway–breathing–circulation–disability–exposure), remembering that an airway obstruction is potentially deadly faster than a respiratory problem which, in turn, can turn fatal faster than a circulatory problem, etc. (Fig. 1.1).

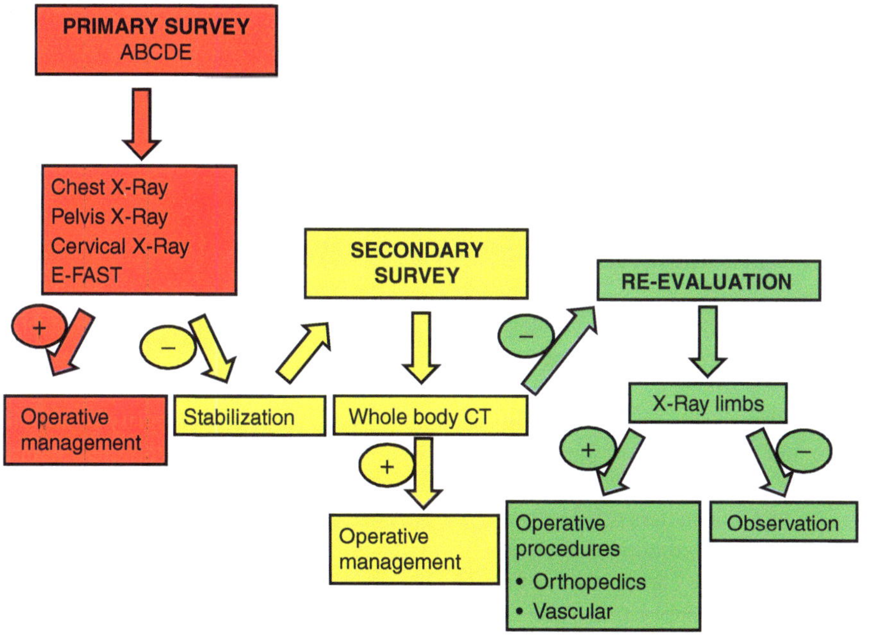

Fig. 1.1 Flow chart

1.2.1 Airway: Airway and Cervical Spine Protection

Ensuring airway patency is the first essential step for the resuscitation of polytrauma children: in fact, an acute airway obstruction is the leading cause of death in pediatric trauma.

Clinical signs of partial or complete airway obstruction are, for example, stridor, dysphonia, wheezes, high or too low respiratory rate, but also – indirectly – altered state of consciousness (restlessness, stupor, coma).

The first fundamental maneuver of the opening of the airway is the jaw-thrust maneuver which allows to maintain the alignment of the cervical spine; at the same time, high oxygen concentration should be administered immediately and a cervical collar should be placed. In children, the dimensional proportion between the head and body, with the typical prominent occiput, requires almost always to raise slightly the trunk in order to allow the cervical spine to stay in-line.

The airway patency may be impaired by the hypotonia of the tongue, hypopharyngeal muscles, as well as by secretions, blood, vomit, foreign bodies, and direct injuries of the facial bones/skull or of the airways.

The final maneuver of "stabilization" of the airway is represented by tracheal intubation to be performed only by skilled care providers.

Basic indications for tracheal intubation are:

- Airway protection from aspiration of blood and vomitus
- Airway obstruction or risk of obstruction due to trauma and burns of the face and/or of the neck
- Insufficient oxygenation despite a high Fi02
- Shock
- Severe impairment of the levels of consciousness (GCS <9)

1.2.2 Breathing: Ventilation and Oxygenation

A consequential step immediately following the verification and obtainment of a patent airway is monitoring the effectiveness of respiration – spontaneous ventilation.

An efficient respiratory activity depends on the anatomical integrity of the rib cage and the pulmonary parenchyma, in addition, of course, to an efficient neural drive.

As in adult patients, it is absolutely necessary to seek and rule out clinically life-threatening conditions such as tension pneumothorax and open pneumothorax, using the classic cornerstones of physical examination: inspection, palpation, auscultation, respiratory rate observation, and Sp02.

Tension pneumothorax still represents a dangerous and unrecognized "killer," responsible for many preventable trauma deaths.

In children and even more in infants, any impairment in diaphragmatic excursion may significantly decrease ventilation. This occurs, for example, in the presence of gastric dilatation due to air ingestion (crying) or involuntary insufflations during ventilation with mask. Therefore, it is always convenient to take into account the decompression of the stomach using a G-tube.

In presence of severe impairment, ventilation is to be assisted with bag-valve mask (BVM) unit or tracheal intubation.

1.2.3 Circulation: Circulation and Hemorrhage Control

Assessment of the pediatric trauma patient's circulation must take into account the peculiar stress and hypovolemia response; thanks to a significant release of catecholamine, the trauma child can compensate for blood loss increasing the heart rate and the systemic resistance; as a result, differently than adults, arterial hypotension is a late sign of shock and it often leads to imminent cardiac arrest.

Assessment of trauma child's cardiovascular status is to be based on a combination of parameters, such as consciousness level, skin appearance (paleness, sweating, mottled skin), capillary refill time (normal <2 s), decrease of peripheral pulse rate compared with the central one, and dieresis (as soon as possible).

The lower arterial blood pressure values, considered acceptable in relation to age, are [11]:

- Newborns, from 0 to 28 days old: 60 mmHg
- Infants, from 1 to 12 months old: 70 mmHg
- Children, from 1 to 10 years old: 70 mmHg + (2 mmHg per each year)

It is always required to identify the presence of any source of external bleeding with a systemic approach, by applying direct pressure; in children, in particular, the bleeding from the skull can be very massive and hemodynamically significant; in the presence of uncontrolled bleeding from the limbs, it required the immediate use of pneumatic tourniquets of proper fit.

All the polytrauma pediatric patients should be connected to a multiparameter monitor in order to have a continuous reassessment of the respiratory and circulatory parameters.

It is essential to obtain, as soon as possible, one or, preferably, two vascular access for the replacement of fluids and the delivery of medications. When a vascular access is unavailable within few minutes, it is suggested the installation of an intra-bone passage in the tibial, femoral, or humeral site (Fig. 1.2) [12].

In case of hypovolemic shock in a pediatric patient, the infusion plan involves the administration of a rapid 20 ml/kg bolus of crystalloids that can be repeated up to three times to a total of 60 ml/kg. If hemodynamic stability is not achieved, then further 10 ml/kg bolus of red blood cell concentrate is to be given. As in adults, also in children, the administration of colloids is highly controversial.

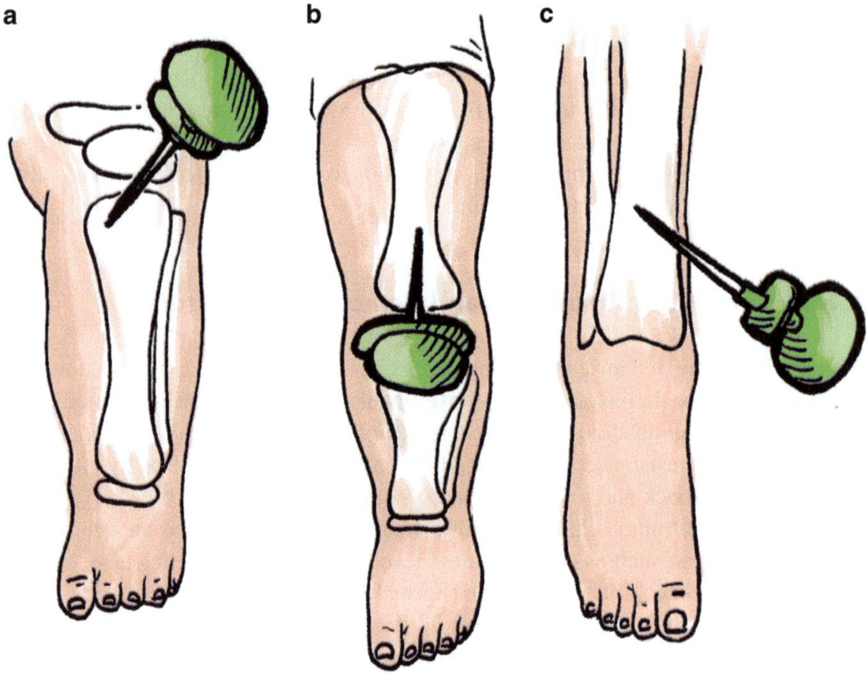

Fig. 1.2 Intra-osseous vascular access (**a**) Proximal tibiae site, (**b**) Femoral site, (**c**) Distal tibial site

It is beyond the present study a detailed survey of the infusion strategies and the relative clinical target in different traumatic situations (head trauma and/or closed and/or penetrating trauma). However, it is important to remember that a careless volemic expansion, above all if performed without heating the fluids, can cause harmful coagulation impairment, from hemodilution and hypothermia.

As in adults, a shock condition in trauma children is to be attributed to hemorrhage, until proven otherwise; in relation to the context, of course, different and concurrent causes should be assessed, such as myocardial dysfunction after contusion due to thoracic trauma or medullary impairment with neurogenic shock (hypotension without increase of heart rate or vasoconstriction) due to head and neck injuries.

1.2.4 Disability: Neurological Assessment

Primary survey is to be completed assessing level of consciousness, papillary size and reaction, and possible lateralizing signs.

The level of consciousness can be examined using the Glasgow Coma Scale (GCS) (Table 1.3) or the simplest score AVPU (Table 1.4).

A modified version of the GCS, the Pediatric Coma Scale (PCS) (Table 1.5), has been studied for preschool children.

Table 1.3 Glasgow Coma Scale

Eyes (1–4 points)	Verbal (1–5 points)	Motor (1–6 points)
4. Opens eyes by himself	5. Oriented (normal)	6. Obeys commands
3. Opens eyes in response to voice	4. Confused (disoriented)	5. Localizes pain
2. Opens eyes in response to pain	3. Says inappropriate words	4. Withdraws from painful stimulus
1. Does not open eyes	2. Makes meaningless sounds	3. Decorticate posturing with painful stimulus
	1. Makes no sounds	2. Decerebrate posturing with painful stimulus
		1. Makes no movements

Table 1.4 AVPU system

A=**a**lert
V=response to **v**erbal stimuli
P=**r**esponds to painful stimuli
U=**u**nresponsive

Table 1.5 Pediatric Coma Scale (PCS)

Eyes (1–4 points)	Verbal (1–5 points)	Motor (1–6 points)
4. Opens eyes spontaneously	5. Coos and or babbles	6. Infant moves spontaneously or purposefully
3. Opens eyes in response to speech	4. Cries but consolable, inappropriate interactions	5. Infant withdraws from touch
2. Opens eyes in response to painful stimuli	3. Inconsistently inconsolable, moaning	4. Infant withdraws from pain
1. Does not open eyes	2. Inconsolable, agitated	3. Abnormal flexion to pain for an infant (decorticate response)
	1. No verbal response	2. Extension to pain (decerebrate response)
		1. No motor response

Among the causes of neurological alterations in a pediatric trauma patient, it is necessary to consider a possible reduced intake of O_2 (respiratory or cardiocirculatory causes) and hypoglycemia (easily exhaustible glycogen stores).

1.2.5 Exposure: Exposure and Thermal Protection

In the last stage of the primary survey, the trauma patient should be completely undressed (rapid external examination) and soon after protected from the risk of thermal dispersion (convective warming system, isothermal blanket).

1.3 Secondary Survey

The secondary survey is the phase of assessment and definitive treatment of the trauma patient.

It is undertaken only after the primary survey has been completed, in condition of total stability of the vital parameters.

It is necessary to act with order, from head to toe.

1.3.1 The Role of Radiology in the Management of Pediatric Polytrauma

Emergency radiology plays a crucial and vital role for the diagnostic iter of a poly-trauma child, but it cannot take the place of a detailed history and a thorough physical examination.

Several imaging techniques are available, each one with its own advantages and its limits (Table 1.6), and the radiologist must be prepared to promptly decide which method to use so as to collect a lot of useful information for physicians and surgeons to develop an appropriate treatment and/or surgical plan.

Radiological examinations may determine waste of valuable time in the poly-trauma management. For this reason, in emergency management, the sensitivity of

Table 1.6 Advantages/disadvantages of imaging modalities [16]

Imaging modality	Advantages	Disadvantages
X-ray	Very accessible	2D images
	Rapid	Artifact from superimposed structures
	Low cost	Limited use for soft tissues
		Ionizing radiation (negligible dose)
Ultrasound	Generally accessible	Operator dependence
	No ionizing radiation	Limited by body habitus
	Low cost	Potentially painful
	Dynamic image capture	Inconclusive results
	Procedural guidance	
	Bedside test	
Computed tomography	Generally accessible	Ionizing radiation
	Rapid	Contrast-induced nephropathy
	High specificity/sensitivity	Intermediate cost
	3D images	Contrast allergy
Magnetic resonance	No ionizing radiation	High cost
	High sensitivity/specificity	Limited availability
	No contrast nephropathy	Long study duration
		May require sedation for children or cause claustrophobia

a radiological investigation is more important than its specificity, with the major aim of excluding any morbid conditions which would require a prompt curative treatment.

In the diagnostic evaluation of a polytrauma patient, the path to follow is completely different depending on whether the patient is in clinical condition of hemodynamic stability or instability.

As a matter of fact, in hemodynamically stable patients or in patients stabilized after primary resuscitation, a whole-body CT scan can be performed for a thorough and detailed exam of all the body parts, both visceral and somatic; on the contrary, in hemodynamically unstable patients, CT scan cannot be performed due to lack of time, and, therefore, lifesaving radiological and ultrasound investigations should have been already performed in the emergency setting, during the primary survey stage [13].

Upon arrival of polytrauma patients at the emergency setting, the radiologist plays a key role in the primary survey, and in this scenario, radiological and ultrasound examinations play a definite role, capable of providing a first effective diagnostic confirmation of some potentially life-threatening clinical situations.

Imaging tests to be performed during this stage are chest X-ray on AP view, cervical spine X-ray on LL view, pelvis X-ray on AP view, and E-FAST scan (extended focused assessment with sonography for trauma) with the patient lying in a supine position while the resuscitators try to monitor and stabilize the pediatric patient's vital signs. The whole-body CT, as already said, on the contrary, a diagnostic aid of the secondary survey, is performed only after the achievement of the hemodynamic stability so as to meet a detailed and complete evaluation of all the body.

This chapter, therefore, will treat in detail only those semiotic elements relating to the investigations with diagnostic aids of the primary survey stage; the technique of whole-body CT scan will be only mentioned. The CT semiotic elements of the injuries of each organ and the whole body will be treated separately in the other specific chapters.

1.3.1.1 Chest X-Ray (CXR)

The CXR study on AP view, at bedside, of the polytrauma patient in the emergency room can be performed in the primary survey of an unstable trauma patient, in the presence of:

(a) Respiratory failure (hypoxemia, dyspnea)
(b) Hemodynamic instability
(c) After pleural decompression or pleural drainage insertion

The diagnostic priorities for these patients are two and are related to the detection of pneumothorax and hemothorax; besides, parenchymal injuries due to more or less extended contusion or lacerations, fractures of the thoracic wall, etc., can be detectable, as well.

1.3.1.1.1 Pneumothorax (PNX)

Pneumothorax affects approximately 60 % of patients with severe chest trauma and can be fatal even in the absence of other organ injuries.

A simple PNX occurs when the pressure of the air in the pleural cavity does not exceed that of the atmosphere; in a tension PNX, on the other hand, such pressure increases because a pleural–parenchymal or bronchial injury acts as a "one-way valve," allowing air to enter but not to escape from the pleural cavity with each ventilation.

Tension PNX is the most severe form of PNX; it can result in a fatal cardiopulmonary failure and it is a common cause of death for chest injury.

The superiority of the MDCT compared to the CXR in the diagnosis of PNX is well known; the radiographic diagnosis of PNX should be considered a difficult diagnosis, and cases of unrecognized PNX on XR and diagnosed only on MSCT have achieved a percentage of 40 % in some studies.

The diagnostic difficulties in recognizing PNX are due to the not always excellent technical qualities of CXR and the specific semeiological characteristics that PNX takes on CXR. In fact, in upright position (orthostasis), the diagnosis of a PNX is based on the identification of the visceral pleura seen tangentially from the radiant beam (pleural line, more remarkable in the external apical/subclavian regions) and the complete absence of pulmonary pattern laterally to the "pleural line"; on the contrary, in supine position (clinostasis), the semeiotics of PNX is completely different, and in fact, the lateral-costal placement of PNX is quite uncommon, as well as the indication of the "pleural line."

This occurs because, with a polytrauma patient in clinostasis:

1. PNX preferably collects in the lower anterior portion of the chest, above all, in the anteromedial and subpulmonary site, where the flap, interposed between the base of the lung and the diaphragm, can locate both at the front and posteriorly. In such cases, the radiant beam does not tangentially detect any visceral pleural border, and the sign of the "pleural line" is not appreciable.
2. The lung presents compliance alterations (contusion, edema) that may prevent a harmonic collapse toward the hilum: the presence of lung pattern external to the supposed "pleural line" does not rule out the diagnosis of PNX.

The radiological signs to detect a PNX in supine position (clinostasis) are (Fig. 1.3):

- Hyperlucency of the lower part of the chest and the upper quadrants of the abdomen
- Lateral deep sulcus sign in the pleural space
- Double diaphragm appearance
- Sharp appearance of the diaphragmatic edge
- Sharpness of the cardio-phrenic fat pad
- Sharpness of the lower surface of the lung
- Direct visibility of the pleural surface of the lung (more frequent in apical position)

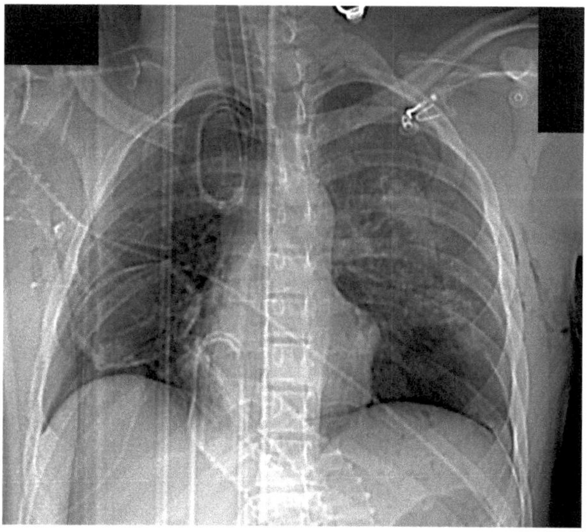

Fig. 1.3 Polytrauma, car crash, transported patient. Left basal pneumothorax, with mantle air flap and thickening of the lung parenchyma. Subcutaneous emphysema of the thoracic wall. Note the hyperlucency of the left lung basis and the deep sulcus sign

Air can, also, separate the edges of the heart, aorta, and vena cava that take an unusual sharp appearance.

It is essential to carefully inspect the lower lobes of the lung and the upper abdomen to avoid misunderstanding such signs. In general, if small amounts of PNX, unrecognized on anterior-posterior view, have no clinical relevance, they may expand rapidly in a patient intubated and under positive-pressure ventilation and may put at risk the patient's life. In such scenario, the radiographic demonstration of rib fractures and homolateral subcutaneous emphysema are to be considered as a sign of PNX, even without sharp intrapleural gas falds.

Tension pneumothorax is an emergency medical condition that requires an immediate treatment, resulting in a reduction of the cardiac filling due to an impairment of the venous blood return and in an alteration of the respiratory exchanges due to the compression of the lung on the ipsilateral and contralateral side.

About 1/3 of patients with unrecognized PNX progress into tension PNX.

The radiographic diagnosis can detect tension PNX through the following signs (Fig. 1.4):

- Contralateral displacement/shift of the mediastinum
- Depression of the diaphragm
- Rib cage expansion
- Flattening of the cardiac profile

The shift of mediastinum is not a specific sign, because it is also visible, to some extent, in simple PNX, whereas the flattening of the cardiac profile is the sign more related to the cardiovascular and respiratory distress that dramatically characterizes the tension PNX. If tension PNX is persistent, despite the correct functioning of drainages, it is essential to rule out any injury of the main airways.

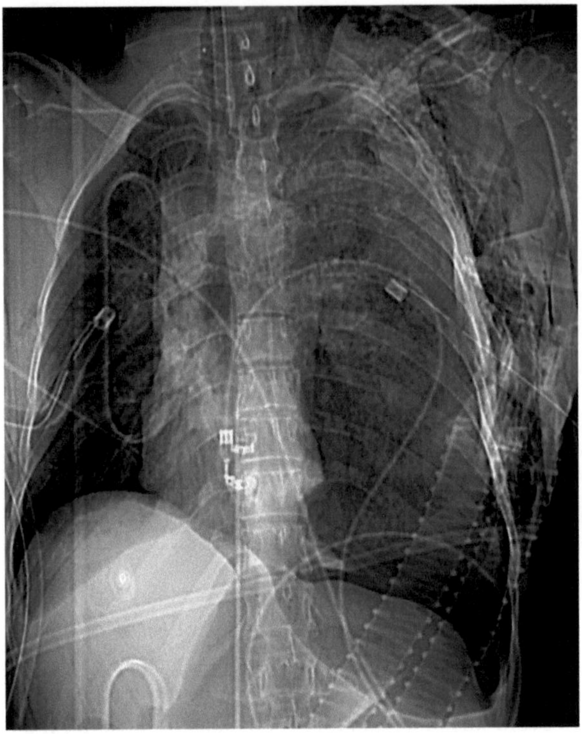

Fig. 1.4 Polytrauma, major dynamics, car against a motorcycle. Left tension pneumothorax, with contralateral dislocation of the mediastinum, lowering of the hemidiaphragm, extension of the intercostal spaces, flattening of the cardiac profile. Large subcutaneous emphysema of the left lateral wall

1.3.1.1.2 Hemothorax

In a blunt chest trauma, pleural effusion is recognizable in about 30–50 % of cases, and in most cases, it can result in hemothorax by laceration of intercostal vessels, pulmonary contusions, and lacerations or injuries to the diaphragm.

The management of hemothorax depends firstly on its initial quantity and the amount of blood flow that it supplies and then on the health condition of the patient; the decisive treatment is, generally, the insertion of a tube thoracostomy.

The initial recesses of the pleural cavity occupied by blood effusion are declivous and variable related to recumbence; instead, with the progressive filling of the pleural cavity, the lateral pleural spaces are invariably involved upward at the apex (apical cap): they are pleural effusions of considerable magnitude, in the order of about 800–1,200 cc.

In orthostatic position, the most declivous part of the pleural space is the subpulmonary space: the classical radiological picture is the visible diaphragm elevation with flattening of its medial profile. When 200 cc of effusion is collected, the meniscus-shaped fluid, visible tangentially from the radiant beam, obliterates the costophrenic angle.

On the other hand, in a supine patient, blood lies posteriorly and along the posterior pleural space; it is acquired on the frontal view on CHR, not tangentially from the radiant beam: for this reason, the formation of meniscus is not always

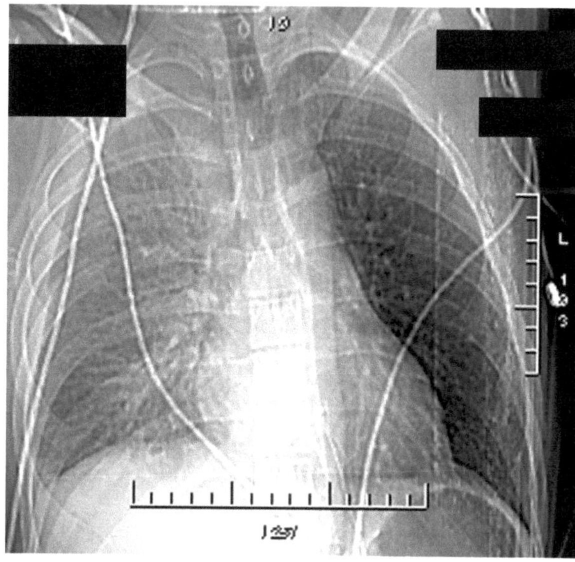

Fig. 1.5 High-energy trauma, scooter against a tree. Right massive hemothorax that presents with large opacity of the entire right hemothorax. Obliteration of the costophrenic angle

detectable, and the radiological sign often shows only a uniform increase of basal-medium density over the hemithorax, through which parenchymal markings appear visible, along with the obliteration of the costophrenic angle (Fig. 1.5). In clinostatic position, effusion lower than 200–300 cc is not usually recognizable, and even massive effusions, placed posteriorly, may be unrecognized.

The contralateral shift of the mediastinum may indicate a hemothorax under pressure, possibly due to arterial bleeding.

1.3.1.1.3 Parenchymal Injuries

Pulmonary contusion is the most common parenchymal injury following the closed chest trauma and, therefore, is the most common cause of pulmonary opacity on CXR, with a prevalence of 30–75 %. It is a hemorrhagic edematous focal deposit, expression of a damage to the alveolar capillary bed in interstitial and endoalveolar site.

The radiographic picture is represented by focal or multifocal areas of confluent "ground-glass" opacity (Fig. 1.6) or consolidation (Fig. 1.7). Contusions do not have segmental boundaries and are usually appreciable in the lung periphery adjacent to the site of trauma.

Contusion may not be radiographically apparent within 6 h of the initial injury but tends to develop gradually in 24–72 h, when they reach their maximum size. In simple clinical cases, contusion shows a progressive reabsorption between 3 and 14 days: opacities that, within this period, have not regressed or rather have enlarged raise the suspicion of developing infection or ARDS.

Pulmonary laceration is a real tear in the lung parenchyma secondary to shearing stress forces ("high-energy" trauma) or direct puncture (bone stumps of rib fracture).

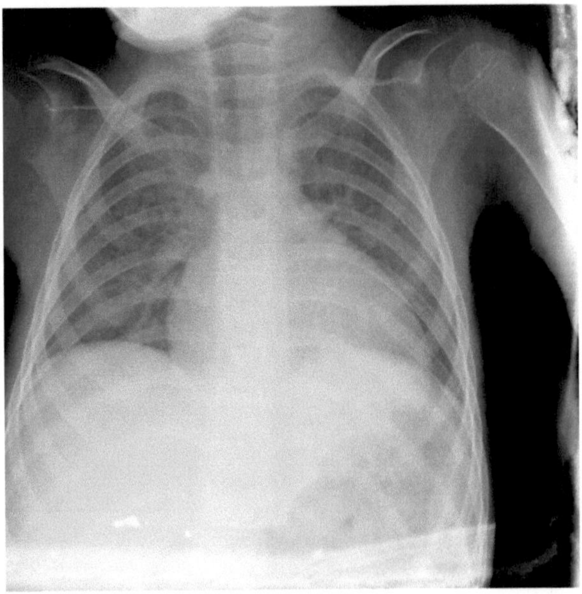

Fig. 1.6 Major trauma, pedestrian, victim of a road accident. Right pulmonary contusion, with confluent unhomogeneous areas of opacity

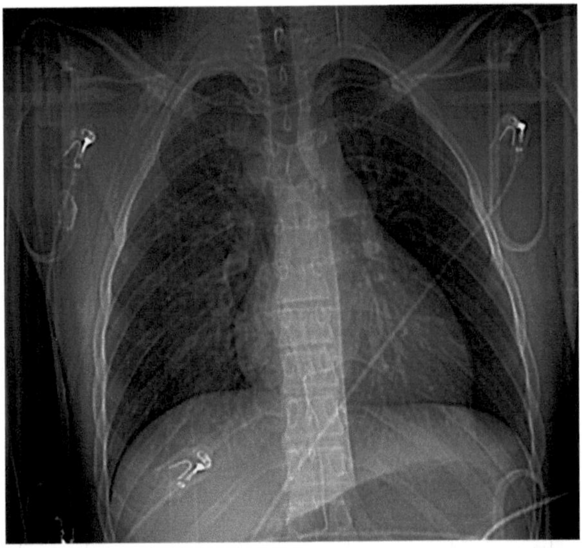

Fig. 1.7 Major dynamic polytrauma, car crash, transported patient. Right pulmonary contusion, with irregular opacity of the parailiac region

On CXR (Fig. 1.8), the radiographic picture is variable: in general, the elastic recoil properties of the surrounding lung results in round-shaped lacerations that are frequently difficult to detect on CXR; however, the picture tends to change in the following inspection.

The space created by the tissue disruption may have air, blood, or more often mixed content, with the formation of air–fluid levels.

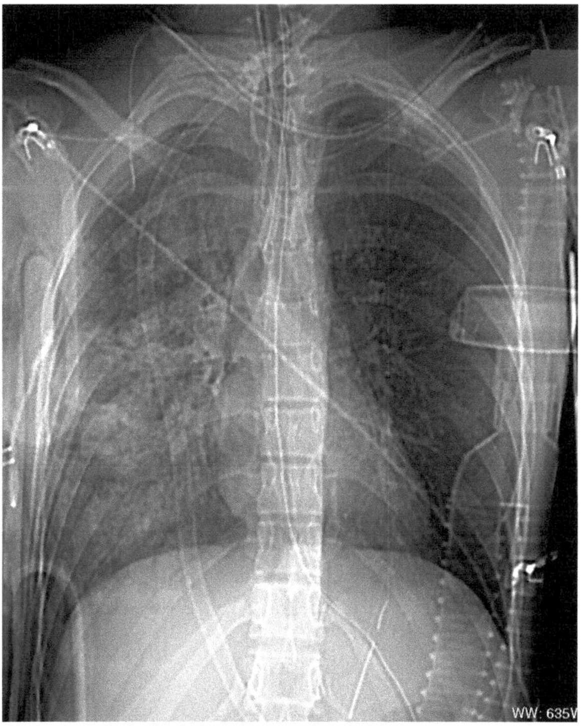

Fig. 1.8 Polytrauma, fall from height. Right large lacerated and contused area, with unhomogeneous parenchymal thickening

Passing the time, the hematoma is reabsorbed and replaced by an elliptical or spherical collection of air, also called post-traumatic pneumatocele (Fig. 1.9). A post-traumatic pneumatocele occurs within few days from the trauma, but in some cases, it may occur after some months; the size is usually between 2 and 5 cm.

Pulmonary atelectasis following a closed trauma may be obstructive (mucus plug, foreign body, endobronchial blood, or airway rupture), passive, compressive, or adhesive.

The diagnosis of obstructive atelectasis is based on the local decrease of air content and of the parenchymal volume: radiographically, subsegmental, segmental, or lobar opacity without air bronchogram, associated with dislocation of the fissures, mediastinum, hilum, and hemidiaphragm of the affected side, may be present.

In obstructive atelectasis, the atelectatic lung may appear as hyperdense rim adjacent to the contusive/lacerative area. In passive atelectasis, the parenchymal opacity may remain substantially normal, for the consensual reduction of air content and locoregional blood content; if bronchial branches are not filled with mucus or blood, the air bronchogram is often appreciable, the same occurs in adhesive atelectasis.

It is important to bear in mind that the different types of atelectasis in a trauma patient are variably associated. Their particularly homogenous, dense aspect associated with diversion of the fissures allows the differential diagnosis of contusion and aspiration.

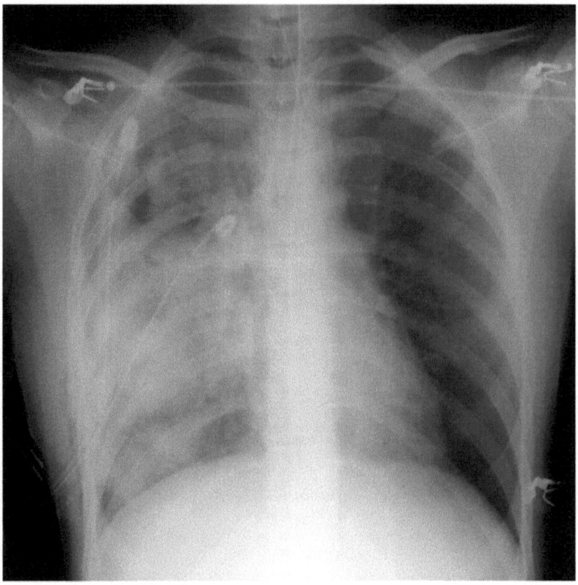

Fig. 1.9 Same patient of the previous figure, development after 48 h. Increase of the opacity in the right lung, related to the increase of blood volume. In the context of opacity appear transparent areas, signs of pneumatoceles

1.3.1.1.4 Vascular Injuries

Traumatic aortic injury is one of the most severe injuries that may occur in "high-energy" polytrauma, with a mortality rate second only to that of traumatic brain injury; moreover, the impairment of vital functions is immediate, and it often occurs directly at the scene of the accident, with an 80–85 % prehospital mortality rate.

If patients are alive upon arrival to the hospital, CXR is the primary screening investigation in the emergency room. The examination is performed in a supine position; it has a sensitivity of 90 % but a poor specificity (25 %) in the detection of mediastinal hematoma.

Visible signs on XR in a supine position on AP view are (Fig. 1.10):

- Signs directly related to traumatic aortic injury: abnormal or indistinct aortic knob contour and/or widening of the aortic knob
- Signs related to the presence of mediastinal hematoma: widening of the upper mediastinum contour, widening of the left paraspinal line, deviation of the trachea or nasogastric tube to the right, depression of the left main bronchus, opacity of the aortopulmonary window, and left apical cap

It is clear that these signs are significantly influenced by the technique of execution of the chest radiogram on AP; moreover, both clinic and radiographic visibility of the injury is more evident in relation to the quantity of the hemomediastinum, the absence of which may be falsely negative.

Therefore, given the high mortality due to aortic rupture and the high risk of vessel injury in high-energy deceleration trauma, every patient with a major deceleration

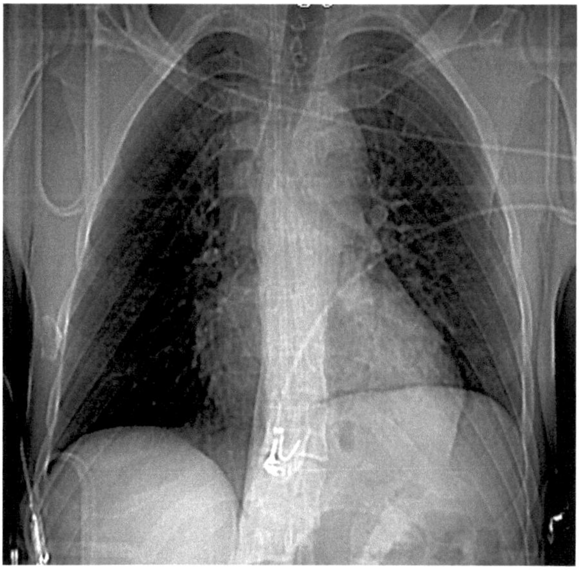

Fig. 1.10 High-energy polytrauma. Aortic rapture and disruption of left hemidiaphragm. The examination in supine position shows the widening of the aortic knob and the right deviation of the trachea. It is also visible the rise of the left hemidiaphragm

trauma should be evaluated with CT scan including contrast medium administration, so as to rule out any traumatic aortic injury.

1.3.1.2 Cervical Spine X-Ray

According to current indications, the X-ray examination of the cervical spine on LL view in a polytrauma patient has been reduced owing to the use of standard protocols that provide for the systematic approach to cervical spine examination with MDCT, during whole-body CT scan.

Furthermore, the cervical spine X-ray on LL view has the advantage to be performed in the resuscitation area without moving the patient and provides relevant information in case of somatic fractures and, above all, vertebral dislocation (Fig. 1.11).

To obtain a complete examination of the cervical spine, effective projections are the anterior-posterior (AP), the latero-lateral (LL), and the AP open mouth for the dens of the axis. In case of need, oblique projections can be added in the study of posterior arch elements.

Radiographs should always be carefully evaluated to search for fractures or vertebral displacements but also to detect abnormalities in vertebral alignment and alterations of the paraspinal and articular soft tissues.

1.3.1.3 Pelvis X-Ray

Fractures of the pelvis have a significant clinical relevance because of the high morbidity and mortality due to frequent complications and associated injuries in other organs or systems (central nervous, respiratory, gastrointestinal, and, above all, genitourinary and vascular systems).

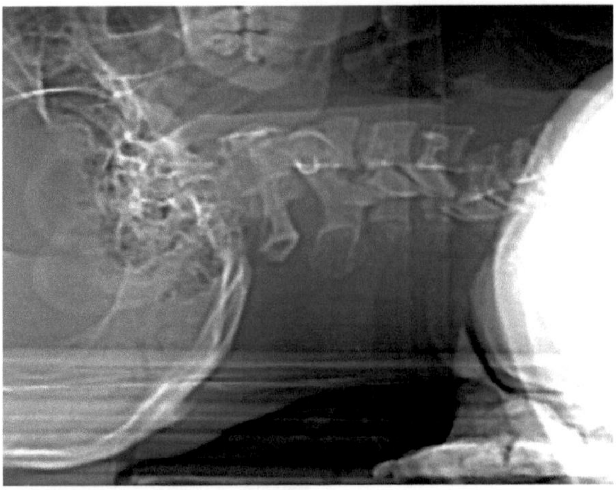

Fig. 1.11 Head and neck trauma due to fall from height (dive in the pool). The projection LL in supine position shows misalignment of the cervical spine, with anterior dislocation of C4 on C5

Management of patient with pelvis fracture depends on the identification of the mechanism of injury and on the degree of pelvic instability.

On the basis of mechanism of injury, fractures are classified as anteroposterior compression, lateral compression, and vertical shear fractures (Fig. 1.12).

The AP projection, recommended by the program ATLS (Advanced Trauma Life Support) performed during the primary survey, provides much information about the mechanism of injury.

Anteriorly, the AP projection allows the identification of the presence and extent of the diastasis of the symphysis pubis and/or the fracture of the obturator ring. Posteriorly, it recognizes the presence and extent of dislocation of the injured side of the pelvis, dislocations of the sacroiliac joint, or fractures of L5 transverse apophysis.

However, this type of projection does not allow to evaluate the real dimension of the injury, especially its posterior component.

Other projections that can add in more information are the following: the oblique outlet view, performed with patient in supine position, caudal-cranial inclination of 30° of the incidental beam centering on the pubis, is useful in quantifying the cranial dislocation of the injured hemipelvis, and the oblique inlet view, performed with patient in supine position, caudal-cranial inclination of 30° of the incidental beam centering on the umbilicus, is useful in documenting the posterior sacroiliac joint dislocation or pubic branches dislocation on AP view, or the inward/outward rotation of the pelvis.

A complete X-ray examination, performed in the ER, is indicated in cases of hemodynamic instability, in the presence of clinically suspected pelvic trauma (unstable fractures, hematuria), in the presence of a suspected hip dislocation, and in the presence of a greater dynamic, if its acquisition does not delay sending a patient in need for an emergency laparotomy in the operating room.

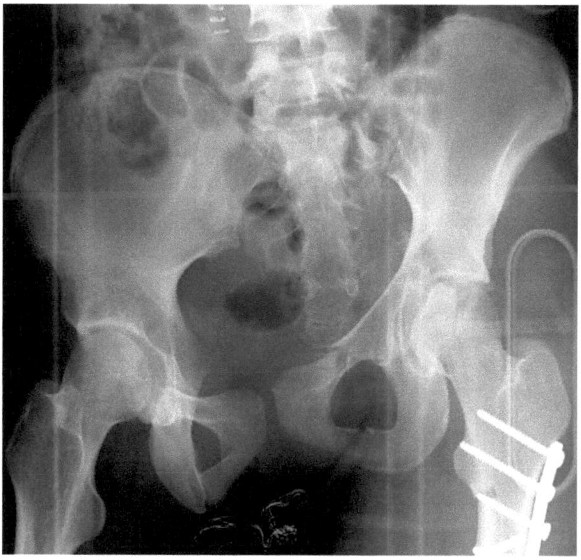

Fig. 1.12 Trauma due to fall from height, patient in his second suicide attempt. Fractures of the left pubic branches, diastasis of pubic symphysis, fracture of the left acetabular bone

1.3.1.4 FAST and E-FAST

1.3.1.4.1 FAST

The use of ultrasound as a lifesaving method in the intensive care unit is now well established according to the protocol FAST (Focus Abdominal Sonography for Trauma), in a polytrauma patient.

The FAST scan is performed at bedside in the ER, usually with a portable machine. Its aim is to identify a free fluid effusion through the ultrasound exploration of the four regions (subxiphoid region, right and left hypochondriac regions, pelvic cavity) (Fig. 1.13).

The FAST scan represents the first level of investigation in finding blood effusions in clinically unstable patients who require a prompt treatment and cannot be moved in the CT unit: it is known from literature that this technique has very high values of sensibility and specificity in the detection of hemoperitoneum (97–100 %) (Figs. 1.14 and 1.15).

However, the classification of abdominal trauma appears partial if the free abdominal effusion is considered as the only diagnostic finding; in literature, it is, in fact, reported that 34 % of patients suffering from parenchymal injuries, also massive, that require a surgical or embolization treatment in emergency may present without abdominal effusion, because the examination is usually performed too early, before the hemoperitoneum becomes visible; finally, the sensitivity of this technique in detecting the hemoretroperitoneum is poor.

In addition, ultrasound has also poor sensitivity in detecting parenchymal traumatic injuries, and practically it has no sensibility in detecting bowel and mesenteric injuries, but they are diagnosable with CT scan.

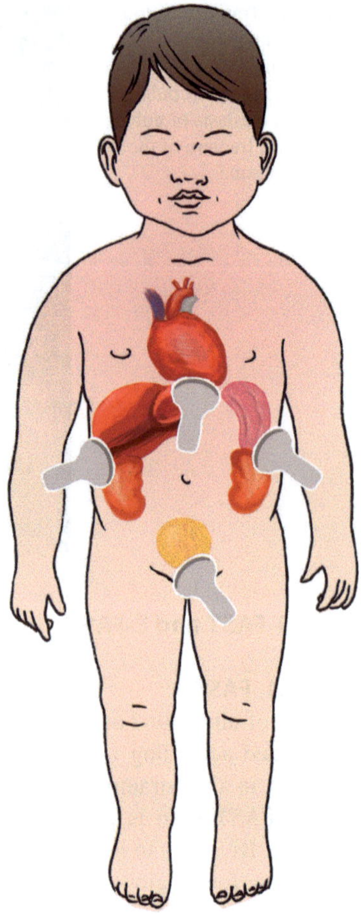

Fig. 1.13 Focused assessment by sonography for trauma (FAST)

Therefore, the effectiveness of ultrasound lies in its high diagnostic accuracy in detecting the hemoperitoneum and in being rapidly performed at the patient's bedside during the primary survey, without hindering resuscitation procedures.

Moreover, in many trauma centers, the FAST scan technique has now been extended, and an E-FAST scan (extended-FAST) is performed for an extension of thorax evaluation.

1.3.1.4.2 E-FAST

The examination of the thorax with the technique E-FAST [14, 15] (Fig. 1.16) aims at identifying the presence of hemothorax (Fig. 1.17) and pneumothorax, including the presence of hemopericardium whose evaluation is already performed with FAST scan, through the execution of some rapid standard scanning with a convex and linear probe (transducer).

PNX air in the pleural space tends to accumulate in the least-dependent part of the chest. This area can be easily located through the observation of the patient and

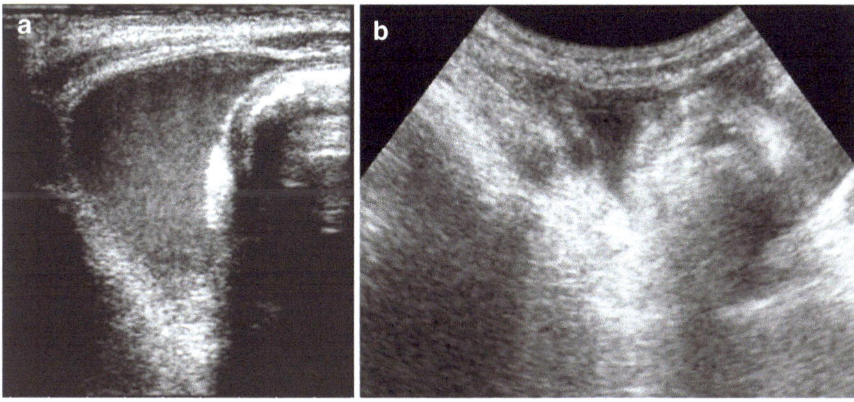

Fig. 1.14 Major trauma, pedestrian victim of a road accident (the same patient in Fig. 1.5). FAST shows hemoperitoneum, with corpuscular effusion in right parietocholeic groove (**a**) and blood collection and blood buildup in pelvic cavity (**b**)

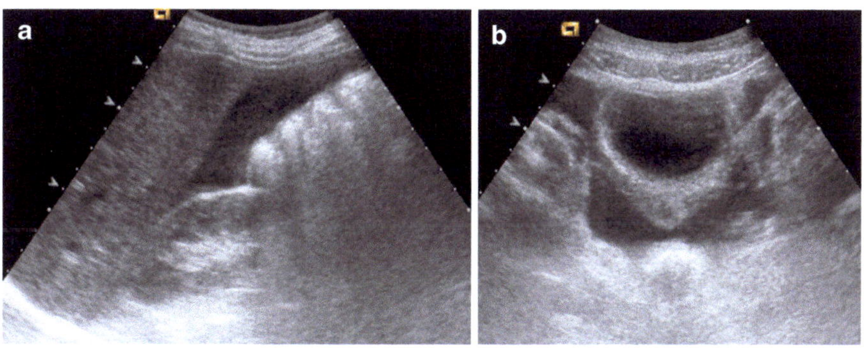

Fig. 1.15 Major trauma, spleen ruptured. (**a**) FAST shows hemoperitoneum, with moderately corpuscular effusion in Morrison's pouch. (**b**) Huge blood volume in the pelvic cavity

the consideration of where any amount of air confined in the pleural space should be placed according to antigravity laws.

When the patient lies in the supine position, the area of interest corresponds to the anterior and inferior part of the chest on both sides of the thorax, approximately the third to fourth intercostal space between the parasternal and the midclavicular lines. This location is easy to scan in almost all inhospital patients, regardless of the clinical condition, patient habits, and respiratory movements. The probe should be gently placed in the intercostal acoustic window of the located area. The parietal pleura appears as a thin echogenic horizontal line located between and below two adjacent ribs. Sometimes, it is necessary to scan more intercostal spaces by moving the probe laterally and inferiorly, in order to evaluate the extension of PNX or to confirm the diagnosis.

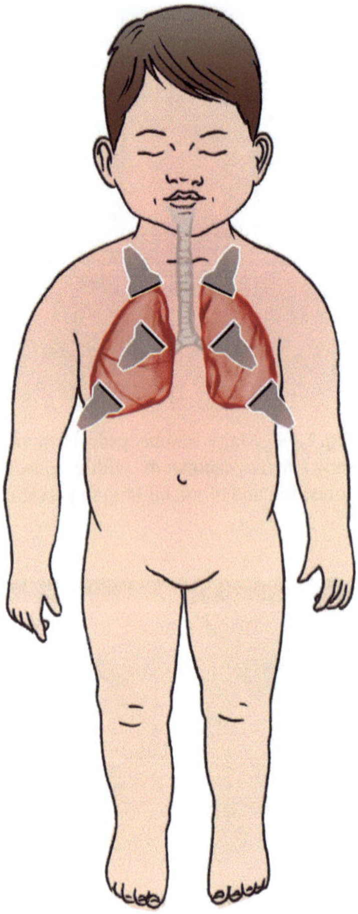

Fig. 1.16 Extended focused assessment by sonography for trauma (E-FAST)

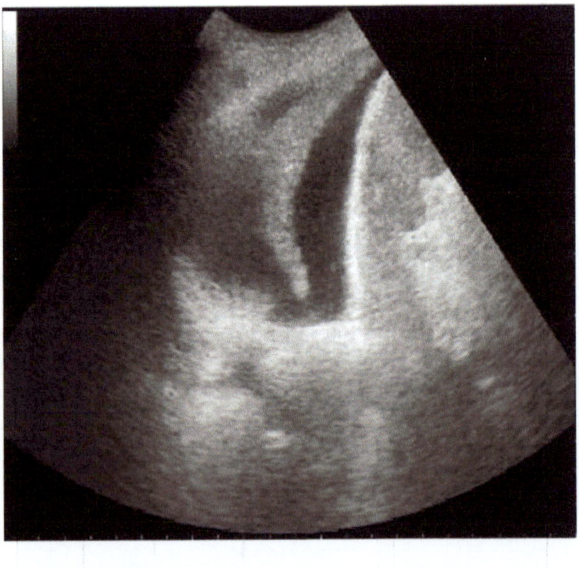

Fig. 1.17 Major trauma. Hemothorax, with corpuscular effusion in the costophrenic pouch. The lower lobe of the lung is atelectatic

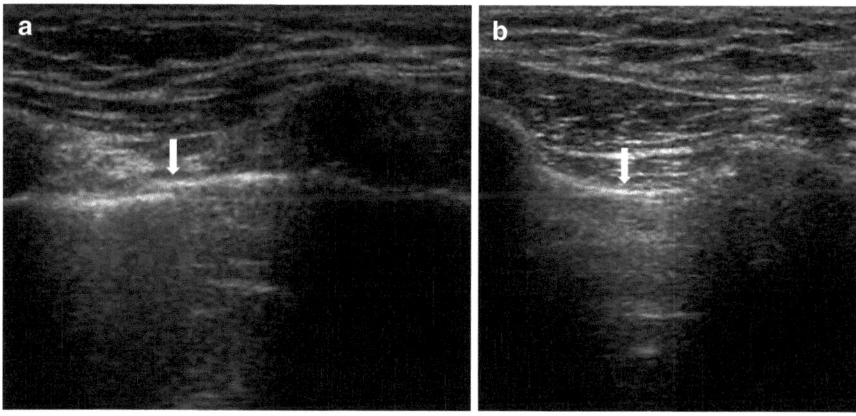

Fig. 1.18 Chest trauma: (**a**) lung point (*arrow*), highly specific sign of pneumothorax; (**b**) only in a dynamic scanning it is possible to notice the presence of pleural sliding, consisting of the sliding of the visceral pleura over the parietal pleura (*arrow*), highly specific sign of pneumothorax absence

The first important dynamic sign to be checked is the "lung sliding." It is a slight and bright horizontal movement of the pleural line which can be checked in a few seconds and is more evident during active and passive respiration. The resolution of the sonograph does not allow distinction between the two pleural layers, and the sliding is an indirect sign indicating the presence of the visceral pleura adhering to the parietal pleura. When air separates the two pleural layers, the movement disappears and cannot be detected by lung ultrasound (Fig. 1.18).

However, the absence of lung sliding does not necessarily confirm PNX, since several other conditions, like massive atelectasis, mainstem intubation, and pulmonary contusion, may cause motionless pleural line. These conditions are particularly frequent in critically ill patients. For these reasons, when LUS is applied in emergency and critical situations, the specificity of absent lung sliding in predicting PNX is reduced (91–78 %).

In an ultrasound evaluation of the lung, the area deep to the pleural line is considered as the artifact zone. Often, some well-defined horizontal or vertical linear echogenic artifact can be visualized. Among the vertical artifacts, the "B lines" are particularly important for the diagnosis of PNX. B lines arise from the pleural line, spread vertically like echogenic rays, reach the lower edge of the screen without fading, and move synchronously with the respiratory movements. These artifacts are the result of multiple reflection of the ultrasound beam between two elements with opposite acoustic impedance, such as the alveolar air and the fluid of the interlobular septa (Fig. 1.19). In PNX, their significance is indirect, because visualization of even one isolated B line represents a safe demonstration of the adherence of the visceral pleura to the parietal pleura. Visualization of B lines rules out PNX with a true negative rate of 100 %. Obviously, the absence of B lines is not a powerful indicator of PNX.

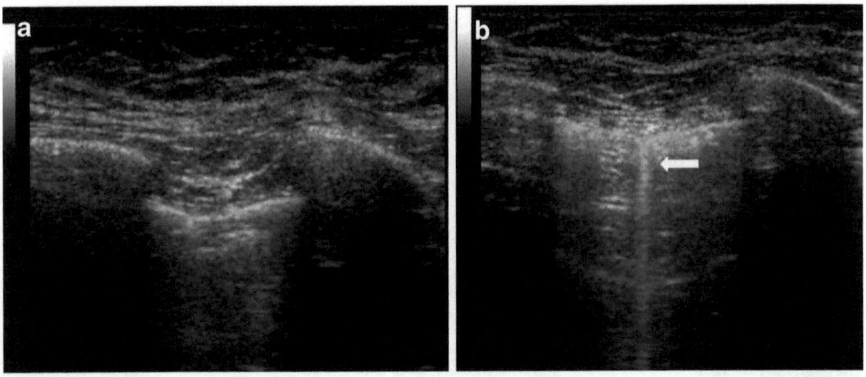

Fig. 1.19 Chest trauma: (**a**) absence of B lines and pleural sliding, presence of pneumothorax; (**b**) presence of B lines (*arrow*). These artifacts are the result of multiple reflection of the ultrasound beam between two elements with opposite acoustic impedance, such as the alveolar air and the fluid of the interlobular septa and they are a sign of absence of pneumothorax

Occasionally, in the absence of lung sliding, a vertical movement of the pleural line synchronous to the cardiac rhythm can be detected. It is called the "lung pulse" and can be caused by the transmission of heartbeats through a consolidated motionless lung. PNX is characterized by the absence of both lung sliding and lung pulse at lung ultrasound because the intrapleural air layer does not allow transmission of both horizontal and vertical movements to the parietal pleura. Thus, visualization of lung pulse rules out PNX.

Contrary to the signs mentioned so far, the lung point allows confirmation of PNX with 100 % specificity. When a sonographic pattern suggestive of PNX (i.e., absent lung sliding and absent B lines) is detected in the anterior-inferior chest area of the supine patients, diagnostic confirmation can be achieved by gradually moving the probe toward the lateral-inferior chest areas. This maneuver is targeted at the detection of a point on the chest wall where a respiratory pattern (i.e., lung sliding and/or B lines) is visualized again and intermittently replaces the motionless pleura. This point is named the "lung point." This is where the lung adheres again to the parietal pleura and corresponds to the lateral edge of the intrapleural air layer.

The presence of abdominal or thoracic free effusion in hemodynamically unstable patients (see previously exposed values) requires an emergency surgical operation.

The presence of pneumothorax requires the insertion of a chest tube directly in the emergency room. A condition of tension pneumothorax could be, in fact, a cause of hemodynamic instability.

If the patients' conditions are good (hemodynamic stability present at the arrival or which occurs after the primary survey), the patient should be suddenly moved to the CT unit to have performed a whole-body CT scan (considered as an integral part of the secondary survey).

1.3.1.5 Whole-Body CT Scanning

In children, CT scan maintains its role as an immediate, pan-scan method with high sensitivity and specificity and less operator dependent compared to the ultrasound.

Although the exposure to ionizing radiation could increase the risk of developing cancer in future life, its immediate and detailed diagnostic accuracy outweighs potential damage.

Even if ALARA's main principle (as low as reasonably achievable) to minimize radiation X-ray exposure in pediatric polytrauma patients has to be always taken into account, the emergency radiologist should not limit the use of a gold standard and potentially lifesaving method for polytrauma children as CT scan [16].

Given the recent advances in technology, a whole-body CT screening can be achieved in a short time, thereby revealing till then hidden injuries and reducing the number of minor injuries that might otherwise be neglected. The whole-body CT scan is the most immediate radiological screening that allows the examination of all the body surface of polytrauma patients.

A single and continuous scan performed from the top to the pubic symphysis allows not only the study of the head, neck, chest, abdomen, and pelvis but also, thanks to the multiplanar reconstruction, the study of the spine, aorta, skull bones, and hips without any further acquisition. These images are quickly done with CT 64-slice with a minimum rotation time of 0.35 s, a maximum table speed of 175 mm/s, and maximum volume coverage of 200 cm. The isotropic design of the 40 mm detector delivers 0.35 mm isotropic resolution and thin-slice (64×0.625 and 32×1.25) imaging in all scan [17].

In pediatric patient, the amount of contrast medium used is highly dependent on the weight. Two milliliter per kilogram is usually given with a speed of injection of 3 ml/s. The injection of a saline solution is always recommended to ensure a compact progression of the contrast bolus (Table 1.7).

1.3.1.5.1 Unenhanced CT Scans

Scans without contrast medium are appropriate for the examination of head and facial mass. The neck, thorax, abdomen, and pelvis are not routinely explored during this stage to prevent an excessive radio-exposure.

1.3.1.5.2 Contrast-Enhanced CT

The contrast-enhanced CT scan includes the examination of the neck, thorax, abdomen, and pelvis. It is generally a multiphase study, with an arterial and a portal venous phase. Only if needed, the study may be completed by a late scan (excretory phase). In whole-body CT scanning, the arterial phase starts from the circle of Willis and extends to the pubic symphysis using the bolus tracking technique with the region of interest (ROI) located in correspondence of the ascending aorta. This phase is important for the study of vascular injuries, such as active bleeding of arterial origin, the presence of post-traumatic pseudoaneurysms, and acute arterial thrombosis (e.g., at the level of the carotid). The portal venous phase includes only the examination of the abdomen, from the diaphragm to the iliac bones. This phase

Table 1.7 Whole-body MDCT protocol in pediatric trauma patients

Unenhanced CT scan	Head, face						
CT+IV cm	Neck, chest, abdomen, pelvis						
	CM concentration	**CM volume**	**Injection rate** (ml/s)	**Delay**	**Rotation time** (s)	**Pitch**	**Detector width** (mm)
16-slice MDCT	300 mg I/ml	2 ml/kg	2–3	Arterial phase: bolus track (ascending aorta)	0.7	1.375	1.25
				Portal phase (abdomen): 40″ after a.p.			
	Saline	30 ml	3	Excretory phase (abdomen) (if necessary): 240″ after p.p.			
64-slice MDCT	350 mg I/ml	2 ml/kg	3	Arterial phase: bolus track (ascending aorta)	0.5	0.938	0.625
				Portal phase (abdomen): 35″ after a.p.			
	Saline	30 ml	3	Excretory phase (abdomen): 240″ after p.p.			

provides relevant information about trauma injuries of the parenchymal organs and the presence of effusion in the peritoneal cavity. The late excretory phase is only required in patients with suspected injuries in the excretory/urinary system (at the renal, pelvic, ureteral, and bladder level) in relation to the presence of a renal injury evident in the portal venous and hematuria phase. The last one is performed 180–240 s after the end of the portal phase, and it shows loss of iodated urine from the urinary system, with the formation of urinomas in the retroperitoneal space or, less frequently, in the peritoneal cavity.

The coronal and sagittal multiplanar reconstructions (MPRs) are routinely performed for the evaluation of the spinal column in the cervical, thoracic, and lumbar regions as well as the evaluation of the thoracic and abdominal structures. The MIPs (maximum intensity projections) and VR (volume rendering) reconstructions are required in case of vascular injuries or fractures of the spine and pelvis.

The use of the whole-body CT scan is rapidly increasing in the management of pediatric polytrauma patients. As mentioned above, we should consider the risk associated with the exposure to ionizing radiation directly related to this technique, but the same, we should carefully consider the cases of cancer and, therefore, of early death directly related with it [18]. In spite of this, the international literature has repeatedly underlined the importance of reducing the radiation dose through mechanisms for modulating the CT [19] beams delivered especially to children and young patients. Although it is prudent to obtain a good image quality to achieve a satisfying diagnosis, it is absolutely required the use of low radiation dose protocols to reduce the number of oncological diseases in future life. Some studies have, in fact, documented that it is possible to reduce the radiation dose compared to that commonly used, maintaining a CT image quality more than satisfying [20].

Low-dose CT protocols have been validated for different regions of the body, including sinuses, facial mass, chest, abdomen, and pelvis.

A weight- and cross-sectional dimension-based adaptation of scanning parameters (tube current and tube potential) has also been recommended to reduce the radiation dose associated with CT scanning [21].

During CT scanning, a user can manually set the scanning parameters to reduce or adjust the radiation dose according to patient size, clinical indications, and body region being scanned. These scanning parameters may include tube voltage, tube current, gantry rotation time, pitch, and beam collimation or detector configuration.

The manual selection of a lower tube current (milliampere) is the most commonly used method to reduce the radiation dose associated with CT scanning [21]. Several studies have demonstrated that low-dose CT with reduced tube current is a useful alternative to standard tube current scanning and can provide satisfactory image quality [22].

References

1. Jaffe D (1991) Emergency management of blunt trauma in children. N Engl J Med 324:1477–1482
2. Minino A, Heron M, Smith B (2006) Deaths: final data for 2004. Natl Vital Stat Rep 54:1–49

3. Peclet MH, Newman KD, Eichelberger MR et al (1990) Patterns of injury in children. J Pediatr Surg 25:85–90
4. Sieben RL, Leavitt JD, French JH (1971) Falls as childhood accidents: an increasing urban risk. Pediatrics 47:886
5. Ablu-Jaude WA (1996) Indicators of genitourinary tract injury or anomaly in cases of pediatric blunt trauma. J Pediatr Surg 31:86
6. Corey TS (1992) Infant deaths due to unintentional injury: an 11-year autopsy review. Am J Dis Child 146:968–971
7. King DR (1985) Trauma in infancy and childhood: initial evaluation and management. Pediatr Clin North Am 32:1299–1310
8. Rutland-Brown W, Langlois JA, Thomas KE, Xi YL (2006) Incidence of traumatic brain injury in the United States, 2003. J Head Trauma Rehabil 21:544–548
9. Sharples PM, Storey A, Aynsley-Gree A, Eyre JA (1990) Avoidable factors contributing to death of children with head injury. BMJ 300:87–91
10. Schafer I, Barkmann C, Riedesser P et al (2006) Posttraumatic syndromes in children and adolescents after road traffic accidents - a prospective cohort study. Psychopathology 39:159–164
11. Kleinman ME, Chameides L, Schexnayder SM et al (2010) Part 14: Pediatric advanced life support: 2010 American Heart Association Guidelines for Cardiopulmonary Resuscitation and Emergency Cardiovascular Care. Circulation 122:876–908
12. Kanter RK, Zimmerman JJ, Strauss RH et al (1986) Pediatric emergency intravenous access. Evaluation of a protocol. Am J Dis Child 140:132–134
13. Miele V, Andreoli C, Grassi R (2006) The management of emergency radiology: key facts. Eur J Radiol 59:311–314
14. Ianniello S, Di Giacomo V, Sessa B, Miele V (2014) First-line sonographic diagnosis of pneumothorax in major trauma: accuracy of e-FAST and comparison with multidetector computed tomography. Radiol Med PMD: 24469989
15. Volpicelli G (2011) Sonographic diagnosis of pneumothorax. Intensive Care Med 37:224–232
16. Baker N, Woolridge D (2013) Emergency concepts in pediatric emergency radiology. Pediatr Clin North Am 60:1139–1151
17. Miele V, Pinto A, Rotondo A (2012) Acute abdomen: rational use of US, MDCT, and MRI. Springer, Berlin/Heidelberg, pp 17–29
18. Ptak T, Rhea JT, Novelline RA (2003) Radiation dose is reduced with a single-pass whole body multi-detector row CT trauma protocol compared with a conventional segmented method: initial experience. Radiology 229:902–905
19. Fanucci E, Fiaschetti V, Totili A et al (2007) Whole body 16-row multislice CT in emergency room: effects of different protocols on scanning time, image quality and radiation exposure. Emerg Radiol 13:251–257
20. Kalra MK, Prasad S, Sain S et al (2002) Clinical comparison of standard-dose and 50% reduced-dose abdominal CT: effect on image quality. Am J Roentgenol 179:1101–1106
21. Kalra MK, Rizzo SMR, Novelline RA (2005) Reducing radiation dose in emergency computed tomography with automatic exposure control techniques. Emerg Radiol 11:267–274
22. Prasad SR, Wittram C, Shepard JA et al (2002) Standard-dose and 50%-reduced-dose chest CT: comparing the effect on image quality. Am J Roentgenol 179:461–465

Paediatric Head Injuries

2

Gianluigi Guarnieri, Anna Nastro, and Mario Muto

2.1 Introduction

Paediatric head injuries (*PHI*) are a common cause for emergency hospital admission all around the world. In North America, head injuries in children occur at an annual rate of 60–100 per 100,000 children [1].

PHI are distinguished as traumatic or accidental brain injury and nonaccidental head injury (child abuse) [2].

Motor vehicle collisions, falls and sport-related accidents are the most common cause of traumatic PHI [2]. Paediatric head trauma can bring about up to 90 % of injury-related deaths, and it includes scalp haematoma and laceration, skull fracture, epi- or subdural haematomas, cerebral contusion, penetrating injuries and diffuse axonal injury (DAI) [2].

Traumatic brain injury (TBI) is defined as 'an alteration to brain function, or other evidence of brain pathology, caused by an external force' by the American Association of Neurologic Surgeons [3, 4].

It results from head injuries, and it is distinguished as minor, mild or severe. Minor TBI has been defined as the child appears neurologically normal and does not present with any symptoms with a Glasgow coma scale (GCS) score of 14–15. Most children sustaining blunt head trauma have minor traumatic brain injury. Mild TBI (GCS score of 13–10) may result in a brief change in mental state or consciousness, while severe (GCS score <10) TBI may result in prolonged unconsciousness, coma or death [5].

Although for the management of severe traumatic TBI clear guidelines are defined including CT and MRI protocol, many controversies remain for minor TBI.

G. Guarnieri • M. Muto (✉)
Neuroradiology Service, Cardarelli Hospital, Naples, Italy
e-mail: gianluigiguarnieri@hotmail.it; mutomar@tiscali.it

A. Nastro
Neuroradiology Service, Santobono Hospital, Naples, Italy

V. Miele, M. Trinci (eds.), *Imaging Trauma and Polytrauma in Pediatric Patients*,
DOI 10.1007/978-3-319-08524-1_2

The aim of this chapter is to try to define the correct imaging management for traumatic PHI, focusing especially on minor head injuries and nonaccidental traumatic head injury.

2.2 Considerations and Guidelines

Cranial CT to detect TBI is obtained liberally in paediatric and adult patients with head trauma because evidence suggests that patients can be safely discharged home after negative findings on CT provided that the patients are neurologically normal [6–8].

Head CT scan is the first imaging tool for the majority of PHI. It is fast, quick and easy to perform with widespread availability. It is considered to be the most valuable neuroimaging test for the acute clinical diagnosis of PHI, detecting different post-traumatic intracranial pathologies: intra- or extra-axial haemorrhagic lesions, cerebral contusion, penetrating injuries and skull fracture. These collections are the same for adults.

According to the *ACR–ASNR Practice Guideline for the Performance of Computed Tomography (CT) of the Brain* [9], CT brain imaging may be performed with a sequential single-slice technique, multislice helical (spiral) protocol or multidetector multislice algorithm. For CT 'standard' of the brain, contiguous or overlapping axial slices should be acquired with a slice thickness of no greater than 5 mm. In the setting of trauma, images should be obtained and/or reviewed at window settings appropriate for demonstrating brain and bone abnormalities as well as small subdural haematomas and soft tissue lesions (subdural windows). For imaging of the cranial base, an axial slice thickness as thin as possible, but no greater than 3 mm with spiral techniques and 2 mm with multidetector and nonspiral techniques, should be used for 2D reformatting or for 3D reconstruction.

A 3 mm thick CT scan from C3 vertebral body (to evaluate the C0–C2 level) to vertex with MDCT-MPR reconstruction with bone windows should be recommended in the paediatric management [9].

The increased use of CT in paediatrics [10], combined with the wide variability in radiation doses, has resulted in many children receiving a high-dose examination adding that cumulative CT radiation exposure incrementally to baseline cancer risk [11].

Radiologists, medical physicists, radiologic technologists and all supervising physicians have a responsibility to minimize radiation dose to individual patients, to staff and to society as a whole while maintaining the necessary diagnostic image quality. This concept is known as 'as low as reasonably achievable (ALARA)' [9, 12].

The low-dose head CT protocol (children with a body mass of less than 20 kg mAs 100, 120 KV; children with a body mass of 20 kg and more mAs 200, KV 120, with an average current-exposure time product of 271 +/− 73) can substantially reduce the amount of ionizing radiation exposure in the paediatric population without compromising the image quality and diagnostic utility [13–15].

The role of MRI in acute PHI is secondary to CT, limited by longer time examination and lesser sensibility for the detection for hyperacute haemorrhage or skull-bone fracture. Anyway, in case of a neurological symptom not completely explained by CT finding, an MRI must be performed. Among all post-traumatic intracranial pathologies, the diagnosis of diffuse axial injury remains more complex. Initially the CT is normal (50–80 %) and MRI is recommended to early detect it. In fact, about 30 % of negative CTs are already positive on MRI [16].

Many guidelines are applied for the CT indication and management of minor, mild and severe TBI based on patient clinical status, trauma history and risk factors.

Among the three different levels of TBI, the management of the minor one remains more controversial. There is considerable disagreement as to the indications for CT in the large number of head trauma cases classified as minor resulting negative [17, 18].

In 2003, the National Institute for Health and Clinical Excellence (NICE) [19] published guidelines for head trauma patients where it was established that an immediate CT head imaging is requested if the following are present:

1. GCS score <13 at any point since injury.
2. GCS score of 13 or 14 at 2 h after injury: request immediate CT head imaging.
3. >1 vomiting episode.

They place emphasis on the use of early CT examinations of the head as opposed to skull radiography and admission for observation, resulting in an increased number of CT head examinations being performed following head trauma. These NICE guidelines are primarily based on an adult population, and the results have been extrapolated to cover children. In paediatrics, any guideline that advocates an increased radiation burden to the population should be questioned and not applied. In order to reduce the radiation exposure for the paediatric population, in 2005 by the Birmingham Children's Hospital [20], new guidelines were published for the use of CT examinations in the child with a head injury. The inclusion criteria for CT admission were as follows:

1. GCS score <13 on hospital assessment (adequate resuscitation must be ensured).
2. GCS score of 13 or 14 2 h following adequate resuscitation.
3. Vomiting: discuss with consultant at >3 vomits or if the child vomits 2 h post-injury.

This protocol could reduce the unnecessary CT for the minor trauma paediatric population.

Comparing to the NICE head injury guidelines would have resulted in a threefold increase in the total number of CT examinations of the head.

Safety concerns, along with issues of cost and practice variability, have led to calls for the development of effective methods to decide when CT imaging is needed.

Clinical decision rules represent such methods and are normally derived from the analysis of large prospectively collected patient datasets, reducing unnecessary CT imaging.

The Canadian Assessment of Tomography for Childhood Head Injury (CATCH) [21] rule was created by a group of Canadian paediatric emergency physicians to support the decision of referring children with minor head injury to CT imaging.

The goal of the CATCH rule was to maximize the sensitivity of predictions of potential intracranial lesion while keeping specificity at a reasonable level [22].

CATCH [21] is a multicenter cohort study, where children with blunt head trauma presenting with a score of 13–15 on the Glasgow coma scale and loss of consciousness, amnesia, disorientation, persistent vomiting or irritability were enrolled consecutively. For each child, the main outcomes were the need for neurologic intervention and the presence of brain injury as determined by CT. Among the 3,866 paediatric patients enrolled, 95 (2.5 %) had a score of 13 on the Glasgow coma scale, 282 (7.3 %) had a score of 14 and 3,489 (90.2 %) had a score of 15. CT revealed that 159 (4.1 %) had a brain injury, and 24 (0.6 %) underwent neurologic intervention. This study assessed a decision rule for CT of the head consisting of high-risk factors:

1. Failure to reach a score of 15 on the Glasgow coma scale within 2 h
2. Suspicion of open skull fracture
3. Worsening headache and irritability

In addition, there are three additional medium-risk factors:

1. Large, boggy haematoma of the scalp
2. Signs of basal skull fracture
3. Dangerous mechanism of injury

The high-risk factors were 100.0 % sensitive (95 % CI 86.2–100.0 %) for predicting the need for neurologic intervention and would require that 30.2 % of patients undergo CT. The medium-risk factors resulted in 98.1 % sensitivity (95 % CI 94.6–99.4 %) for the prediction of brain injury by CT and would require that 52.0 % of patients undergo CT.

In 2009, the Scottish Intercollegiate Guidelines Network (SIGN) [23] has published guidelines for the management of children with head injuries focused on (a) the utilization of radiological imaging, (b) referral for neurosurgical review and (c) post-discharge follow-up. Immediate CT scanning should be done in a child (<16 years) who has any of the following features:

1. GCS score ≤13 on admission
2. Witnessed loss of consciousness >5 min
3. Focal neurological deficit
4. Signs of a basal skull fracture
5. Involved in a high-speed road traffic accident

A CT scan should be considered within 8 h if any of the following features are present:

1. Three or more discrete episodes of vomiting
2. Post-traumatic seizure

3. Clinical suspicion of a nonaccidental injury
4. Amnesia (anterograde or retrograde) lasting >5 min

The management of a mild trauma patient with a brief change in mental state or consciousness, or severe TBI with prolonged unconsciousness or coma, requires an immediate CT scan and then an MRI in order to detect DAI [5].

No specific guidelines are published for the management of 'birth trauma' or 'perinatal trauma'. They include injuries occurring during labour or delivery, caused by mechanical factors. Despite the improvement of obstetric-developed manoeuvres, these events still occur quite frequently. Thanks to its blood specificity, the CT scan is mandatory in the evolution of newborn suffering from birth trauma or perinatal trauma [16].

Extracranial haemorrhage with caput succedaneum or subgaleal haemorrhage or cephalohaematoma can be caused during the delivery. Intracranial haemorrhage is less frequent than the extracranial one, and subdural haematoma at the tentorium, falx or convexity are usually associated with prolonged and traumatic delivery [16].

Nonaccidental head injury in children (NAHI) [24], most often due to abusive head trauma (AHT), is not uncommon and carries a high risk of mortality and morbidity.

AHT involves an inflicted injury to the head and its contents including injuries caused by shaking and blunt impact. The term 'shaken baby syndrome' (SBS) is commonly used to describe one form of abusive head trauma [24].

Vigorous shaking, with or without directly impacting the skull, is the postulated mechanism of injury to the brain or calvarium. Forceful shaking of an infant creates an angular acceleration–deceleration force that can stretch and tear cortical veins that course to the dural venous sinuses through the subarachnoid space and results in haemorrhage into either the subdural or subarachnoid spaces. Axons coursing from grey to white matter or to areas of denser packing may also be stretched and torn, resulting in diffuse axonal or shear injury [24].

Imaging plays an important role in evaluating infants or children referred for accidental or nonaccidental head injury [25]. Non-contrast CT is the first exam for the evaluation of the child with suspected head injury from trauma. Different CT findings can be used as differential diagnosis of accidental or nonaccidental head injury [16]. Scalp haematomas, linear skull fracture, depressed or comminuted skull fracture, epidural haematoma, homogeneous hyperdense subdural haematoma, subarachnoid haemorrhage or cortical contusion have been seen as the most common collections of accidental head injury. Heterogeneous or mixed-density subdural haematoma is the most frequent finding in cases of NAHI due to repetitive episodes of head injury over time but may be observed within 48 h of accidental head trauma. The mixed-density SDH on non-contrast CT reflects the combination of high-attenuation blood from acute haemorrhage or clot retraction and lower-density fluid from unclotted blood, serum or CSF. Interhemispheric subdural haematoma is not specific for inflicted head injury [16, 25].

Retinal haemorrhages [26] are seen more often in NAHI in children and often are bilateral involving the preretinal layer, covering the macula and extending to the periphery of the retina. It is hypothesized that with rotational acceleration of the ocular globe, traction on the retina by the firmly attached vitreous can lead to retinal haemorrhage, folds and separation. Unilateral RHs can be seen in children with accidental head injury. Children with abusive head injury are more likely to present with abnormal mental status and seizures, whereas children with accidental head injury were more likely to have scalp haematomas [26].

Such characteristics may be useful to distinguish accidental from abusive head trauma in children [16, 26, 27]. The MRI is the modality of choice to identify cortical contusion or DAI [16, 27].

2.3 Skull Fractures

An x-ray film should be obtained in all children under 2 years of age with suspected injury in order to detect fractures because of the high probability of nonaccidental injury [28]. Anyway, a CT scan is recommended in case of suspected injury, especially when symptoms or signs of possible neurological injury are present, and also to detect other associated traumatic lesions [29].

The target is to detect the presence of fracture, its location and type and the presence of other lesions associated, for example, with intra- or extracranial haematoma. Fractures can be simple linear, midline, occipital, multiple, complex, diastatic or depressed fractures (Fig. 2.1).

They are more common patterns in nonaccidental cranial trauma, and each of these collections should be specified [30, 31].

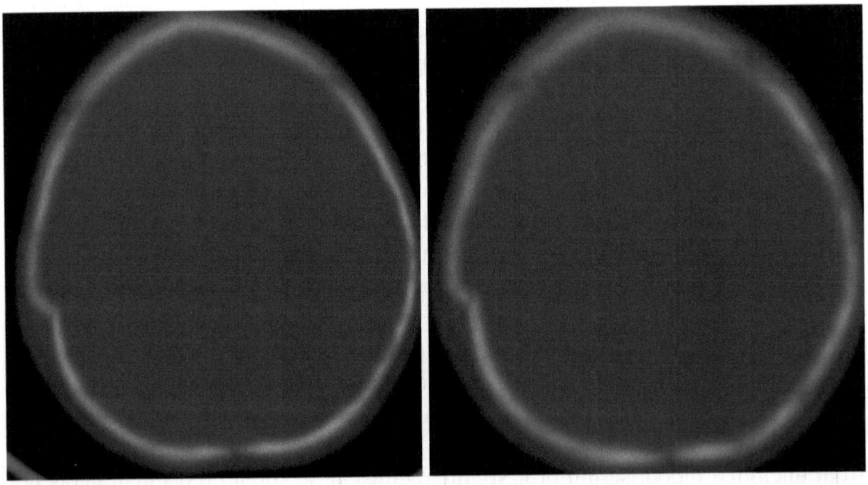

Fig. 2.1 The axial head-MDCT with bone window shows a depressed fracture of the right fronto-parietal bone

2.3.1 Epidural Haematoma

Epidural haematoma (EDH) is secondary to the laceration of meningeal vessels (arteries or veins), diploic veins or dural sinuses in head injuries [32].

Blood extravasates into the virtual epidural space between the inner tabula of the skull and the dura mater. In 90 % of cases, a skull fracture can be associated with it. EDH can be of arterial or venous origin. The arterial one comes out from middle meningeal artery laceration, while the venous one results from dural sinus laceration or diploic veins, and it is more frequent in posterior fossa injury adjacent to the dural sinus especially when a fracture transverses the involved dural sinus. Arterial EDH is typical in older children, while venous EDH is more frequently seen among younger children [32].

On CT, a biconvex-shaped hyperdense finding is the typical pattern of acute EDH due to the pulling away of the dura mater, attached to the skull, by the haematoma (Figs. 2.2, 2.3 and 2.4).

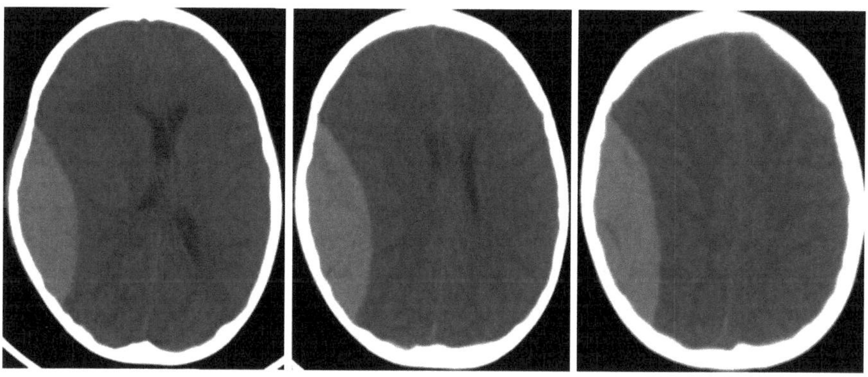

Fig. 2.2 The axial head-MDCT shows a biconvex-shaped hyperdense pattern at the right fronto-parietal region as a typical pattern of acute EDH

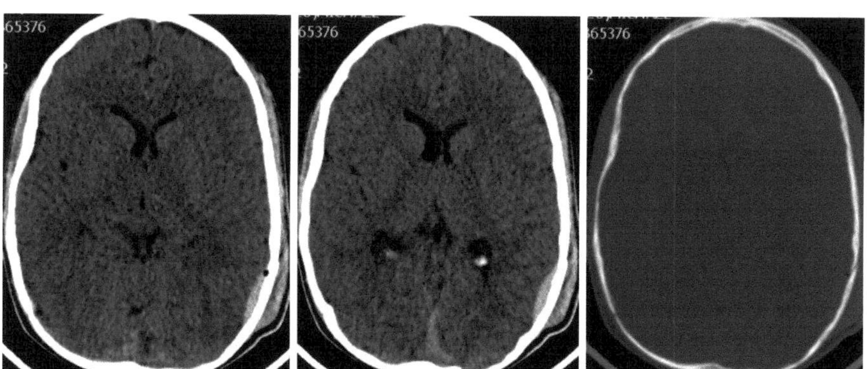

Fig. 2.3 The axial head-MDCT shows a thin biconvex-shaped hyperdense EDH at the left parietal region associated with simple linear fracture of the adjacent bone

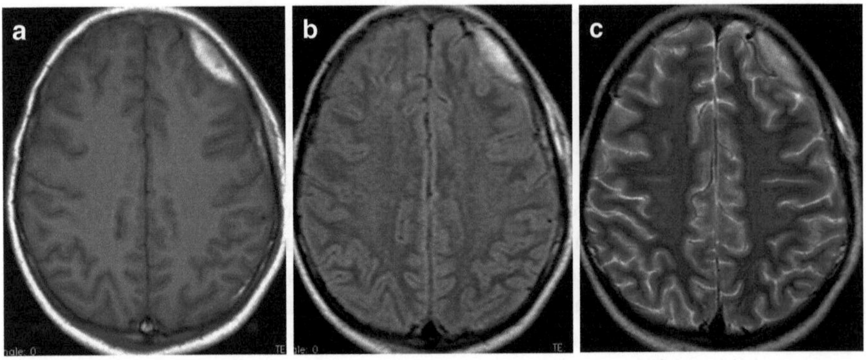

Fig. 2.4 (**a–c**) The MRI shows a left frontal EDH, hyperintense signal on T1W-MRI (**a**), FLAIR (**b**), T2W (**c**) as EDH with extracellular maetaemoglombin signal

Generally, it does not cross the cranial sutures because the periosteal layer of the dura is tightly adherent to the cranial sutures. This sign is used to distinguish EDH from SDH on CT or MRI. By a retrospective data analysis, Huismann [32] showed that in 11 % of children, EDH can cross the cranial sutures especially when fractures involve cranial sutures or when there is a post-traumatic cranial suture diastasis.

Retroclival epidural haematoma may be associated with ligamentous injury, which may further result in instability at the craniocervical junction [33].

2.3.2 Subdural Haematoma

Subdural haematoma (*SDH*) is an extracerebral haemorrhage secondary to torn cortical vein or sinus in head injuries. Blood extravasates into the 'subdural space' which is a potential space that can be opened by the separation of the arachnoid mater from the dura mater as a result of trauma.

Acute (1–5 days) haematomas appear hyperdense (relative to grey matter), whereas subacute (approximately 7–20 days) haematomas appear isodense and chronic (older than 20 days) haematomas hypodense [30].

Accurate timing of a haematoma is not possible after 1 week. The use of intravenous contrast has been recommended to confirm the chronicity of the subdural haematoma by demonstrating the presence of an inner membrane delineating the haematoma [34].

The subdural membrane may be seen after 7 days. A mixed high- and low-density subdural haematoma, representing a chronic haematoma with re-haemorrhage, is considered as a nonaccidental cranial trauma in children (child abuse) [30].

A small extra-axial haematoma or fluid collection can be missed on CT; therefore, MRI is always indicated for detection, thanks to its higher anatomical resolution and multiplanar capability. On MRI, SDH patterns follow the pattern of the evolution of intraparenchymal haematomas in terms of time course. In the acute phase (1–3 days), the signal intensity alteration is a low signal on T1 and on T2.

In the early (3–7 days) subacute phase, the haematoma returns a high signal on T1 and a low signal on T2. In the late subacute (7–21 days) phase, the haematoma returns a high signal on T1 and on T2. In the chronic stage, subdural haematomas may mimic a hygroma by returning a signal similar to that of cerebrospinal fluid on T1 and T2.

A retroclival subdural haematoma may indicate a sentinel event for traumatic injury elsewhere within the brain or posterior fossa [33].

2.3.3 Traumatic Subarachnoid Haemorrhage

Traumatic subarachnoid haemorrhage (tSAH) is defined as a haemorrhage into the subarachnoid space, and it is considered as a marker of severe TBI with adverse outcome [35].

TSAH is caused by the traumatic rupture of small vessels in the pia-arachnoid when the brain is moved under the dura mater by external force during injuries or by haemorrhage associated with cortical contusions. TSAH in the basal subarachnoid cisterns has been considered to indirectly indicate primary brainstem injury in many patients [36].

On CT, the TSAH pattern is a spontaneous hyperdensity into the subarachnoid space or into the basal subarachnoid or sellar cisterns and Sylvian fissures. The degree of TSAH could be classified into three grades according to the density on CT scans: mild, with a faint layer of blood; moderate, with a thin layer of blood; and massive, with a thick layer of blood.

A small amount of blood into the subarachnoid space could be missed on CT scan, but using MRI with FLAIR sequence can detect TSAH [37].

Analysis of the detection of haemorrhagic localizations shows an accuracy, sensitivity and specificity of 89, 82 and 92 % using CT and 90, 83 and 94 % using MRI, respectively. MRI was more sensitive than CT in the detection of subarachnoid haemorrhagic localizations, whereas no significant difference resulted from the detection of epidural and subdural haemorrhagic findings [37].

2.3.4 Brain Oedema

Brain oedema (*BO*) is a bad prognostic sign and usually results in cerebral dysfunction. It can be reversible as long as there is no brain shift or vessel occlusion or can lead to ischaemia.

There are two typical findings for BO: the 'reversal sign' and the 'white cerebellum sign'.

The 'reversal sign' is the diffuse loss of grey–white matter differentiation with decreased attenuation of the cortex. The basal ganglia, cerebellum, thalami and brainstem are relatively spared and may therefore appear relatively bright [38, 39].

The 'white cerebellum sign' reflects the loss of differentiation between cerebral grey and white matter with a loss of density and the sparing of brainstem and cerebellum which may look hyperdense. Often this can also reflect an extracranial non-accidental cause of hypoxia such as strangling or suffocation [38, 39].

2.3.5 Diffuse Axonal Injury

Shear brain injury or more commonly known as diffuse axonal injury (DAI) is diagnosed in children with TBI due to high-impact accident. It is one of the most common and important pathologic features of traumatic brain injury. The susceptibility of axons to mechanical injury appears to be due to both their viscoelastic properties and their high organization in white matter tracts. Although axons are supple under normal conditions, they become brittle when exposed to rapid deformations associated with brain trauma. Accordingly, the rapid stretch of axons can damage the axonal cytoskeleton resulting in a loss of elasticity and impairment of axoplasmic transport. Subsequent swelling of the axon occurs in discrete bulb formations or in elongated varicosities that accumulate transported proteins. Calcium entry into damaged axons is thought to initiate further damage by the activation of proteases. Ultimately, swollen axons may become disconnected and contribute to additional neuropathologic changes in brain tissue. DAI may largely account for the clinical manifestations of brain trauma. However, DAI is extremely difficult to detect noninvasively and is poorly defined as clinical syndrome [40].

DAI is a diagnosis of exclusion whereby the patient who came with a definite history of trauma has a low GCS at presentation but yet a 'normal' brain CT or just multiple small punctate haemorrhages. MRI is a more reliable modality to detect this type of axonal damage instead of CT that is often negative for lesions [41].

DAI can be distinguished in non-haemorrhagic or haemorrhagic lesions.

Non-haemorrhagic ones can be depicted on FLAIR and diffusion-weighted sequences as a small parenchymal subcortical hyperintensity alteration [42] (Fig. 2.5).

In contrast, the haemorrhagic lesions can be detected using T2*-weighted gradient-echo showing very small subcortical microbleeds [43].

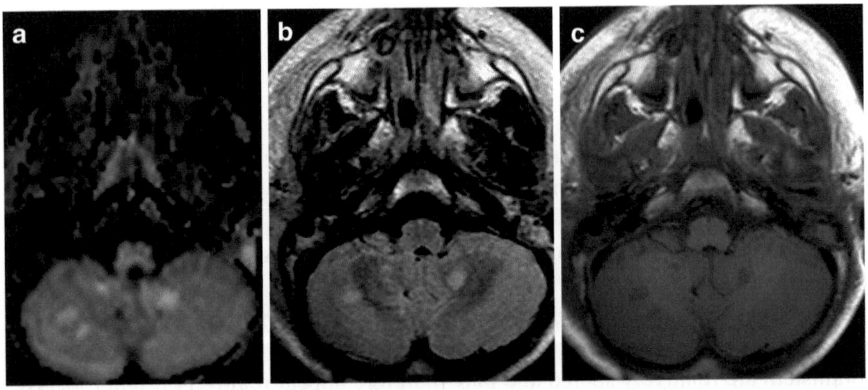

Fig. 2.5 (**a–c**) The MRI shows multiple and small cerebellar subcortical hyperintensity alteration on DWI (**a**), FLAIR (**b**) and hypointensity on T1W (**c**), bilaterally, as posterior fossa DAI

2.4 Conclusions

In the paediatric age, the evaluation of head trauma and head injuries requires clinical criteria for deciding on the type of instrumental diagnostic approach to be made. It needs to emphasize the importance of reducing the use of CT to avoid unnecessary doses to paediatric patients using a low-dose protocol.

CT is the first tool in the acute phase, while MRI is recommended in the subacute phase or follow-up.

References

1. Canadian Institute for Health Information. Head injuries in Canada: a decade of change (1994–1995 to 2003–2004). Available at: http://secure.cihi.ca/cihiweb/en/downloads/analysis ntr 2006 e.pdf. Accessed 10 Apr 2009
2. Atabaki SM (2007) Pediatric head injury. Pediatr Rev 28:215
3. Chan V, Thurairajah P, Colantonio A (2013) Defining traumatic brain injury in children and youth using international classification of diseases version 10 codes: a systematic review protocol. Syst Rev 2:102
4. Brain Injury Association of America: BIAA Adopts New TBI Definition. http://www.biausa.org/announcements/biaa-adopts-new-tbi-definition
5. Thompson MC, Wheeler KK, Shi J, Smith GA, Groner JI, Haley KJ, Xiang H (2014) Surveillance of paediatric traumatic brain injuries using the NEISS: choosing an appropriate case definition. Brain Inj 28(4):431–437
6. Shackford SR, Wald SL, Ross SE et al (1992) The clinical utility of computed tomographic scanning and neurologic examination in the management of patients with minor head injuries. J Trauma 33(3):385–394
7. Livingston DH, Loder PA, Koziol J, Hunt D (1991) The use of CT scanning to triage patients requiring admission following minimal head injury. J Trauma 31(4):483–489
8. Stein SC, Ross SE (1990) The value of computed tomographic scans in patients with low-risk head injuries. Neurosurgery 26(4):638–640
9. ACR–ASNR practice guideline for the performance of Computed Tomography (CT) of the brain. www.asnr.org
10. Miglioretti DL, Johnson E, Williams A, Greenlee RT, Weinmann S, Solberg LI, Feigelson HS, Roblin D, Flynn MJ, Vanneman N, Smith-Bindman R (2013) The use of computed tomography in pediatrics and the associated radiation exposure and estimated cancer risk. JAMA Pediatr 167(8):700–707
11. Sodickson A, Baeyens PF, Andriole KP, Prevedello LM, Nawfel RD, Hanson R, Khorasani R (2009) Recurrent CT, cumulative radiation exposure, and associated radiation-induced cancer risks from CT of adults. Radiology 251(1):175–184
12. Shah NB, Platt SL (2008) ALARA: is there a cause for alarm? Reducing radiation risks from computed tomography scanning in children. Curr Opin Pediatr 20(3):243–247
13. Morton RP, Reynolds RM, Ramakrishna R, Levitt MR, Hopper RA, Lee A, Browd SR (2013) Low-dose head computed tomography in children: a single institutional experience in pediatric radiation risk reduction: clinical article. J Neurosurg Pediatr 12(4):406–410
14. Huda W, Chamberlain CC, Rosenbaum AE, Garrisi W (2001) Radiation doses to infants and adults undergoing head CT examinations. Med Phys 28(3):393–399
15. Jończyk-Potoczna K, Frankiewicz M, Warzywoda M, Strzyżewski K, Pawlak B (2012) Low-dose protocol for head CT in evaluation of hydrocephalus in children. Pol J Radiol 77(1):7–11

16. Tortora Donati P, Rossi A, Biancheri R (2005) Accidental head trauma. In: Tortora Donati P (ed) Pediatric neuroradiology brain. Springer, Berlin, Heidelberg, New York, pp 893–927
17. Stein SC, Ross SE (1992) Mild head injury: a plea for routine early CT scanning. J Trauma 33:11–13
18. Advanced trauma life support for doctors; student course manual, 8th ed (2008) American College of Surgeons, Chicago. American Academy of Pediatrics, Committee on Quality Improvement (1991) The management of minor closed head injury in children. Pediatrics 104:1407–1415
19. Sharavat BP, Huseyin TS, Hynes KA (2004) NICE guideline for the management of head injury: an audit demonstrating its impact on a district general hospital, with a cost analysis for England and Wales. Emerg Med J 21:420e5
20. Willis AP, Latif SA, Chandratre S, Stanhope B, Johnson K (2008) Not a NICE CT protocol for the acutely head injured child. Clin Radiol 63(2):165–169
21. Osmond MH, Klassen TP, Wells GA, Correll R, Jarvis A, Joubert G et al (2010) CATCH: a clinical decision rule for the use of computed tomography in children with minor head injury. CMAJ 182:341–348
22. Klement W, Wilk S, Michalowski W, Farion KJ, Osmond MH, Verter V (2012) Predicting the need for CT imaging in children with minor head injury using an ensemble of Naive Bayes classifiers. Artif Intell Med 54(3):163–170
23. Coulter IC, Brennan PM, Duthie G, Baxter A, McCabe AJ (2011) Are we following the guiding SIGN when managing paediatric head injury? Surgeon 9(2):83–87
24. Roujeau T, Mireau E, Bourgeois M (2013) Nonaccidental head injury. Handb Clin Neurol 112:905–912
25. Tung GA, Kumar M, Richardson RC, Jenny C, Brown WD (2006) Comparison of accidental and non-accidental traumatic head injury in children on noncontrast computed tomography. Pediatrics 118(2):626–633
26. Bechtel K, Stoessel K, Leventhal JM, Ogle E, Teague B, Lavietes S, Banyas B, Allen K, Dziura J, Duncan C (2004) Characteristics that distinguish accidental from abusive injury in hospitalized young children with head trauma. Pediatrics 114(1):165–168
27. Bernardi B, Bartoi C (2005) Nonaccidental head injury (child abuse). In: Tortora Donati P (ed) Pediatric neuroradiology brain. Springer, Berlin, Heidelberg, New York, pp 929–949
28. Lloyd DA, Carty H, Patterson M, Butcher CK, Roe D (1997) Predictive value of skull radiography for intracranial injury in children with blunt head injury. Lancet 349:821–824
29. Minagorre PJ, Aranaz AJ, Flores Serrano J, García AL, Herrero GA (2004) Diagnostic utility of radiography in head trauma: a critical review of the literature. An Pediatr (Barc) 60(6):561–568
30. Demaerel P, Casteels I, Wilms G (2002) Cranial imaging in child abuse. Eur Radiol 12(4):849–857
31. Ochalski PG, Adamo MA, Adelson PD, Okonkwo DO, Pollack IF (2011) Fractures of the clivus and traumatic diastasis of the central skull base in the pediatric population. J Neurosurg Pediatr 7(3):261–267
32. Huisman TA, Tschirch FT (2009) Epidural hematoma in children: do cranial sutures act as a barrier? J Neuroradiol 36(2):93–97
33. Koshy J, Scheurkogel MM, Clough L, Huisman TA, Poretti A, Bosemani T (2014) Neuroimaging findings of retroclival hemorrhage in children: a diagnostic conundrum. Childs Nerv Syst 30(5):835–839
34. Harwood-Nash DC (1992) Abuse to the pediatric central nervous system. AJNR Am J Neuroradiol 13:569–575
35. Armin SS, Colohan AR, Zhang JH (2006) Traumatic subarachnoid hemorrhage: our current understanding and its evolution over the past half century. Neurol Res 28(4):445–452
36. Shigemori M, Tokutomi T, Hirohata M, Maruiwa H, Kaku N, Kuramoto S (1990) Clinical significance of traumatic subarachnoid hemorrhage. Neurol Med Chir 30(6):396–400

37. Añon J, Remonda L, Spreng A, Scheurer E, Schroth G, Boesch C, Thali M, Dirnhofer R, Yen K (2008) Traumatic extra-axial hemorrhage: correlation of postmortem MSCT, MRI, and forensic-pathological findings. J Magn Reson Imaging 28(4):823–836
38. Han BK, Towbin RB, de Courten-Myers G, McLaurin RL, Ball WS (1990) Reversal sign on CT: effect of anoxic/ischemic cerebral injury in children. Am J Roentgenol 154:361
39. Rao P, Carty H, Pierce A (1999) The acute reversal sign: comparison to medical and non-accidental injury patients. Clin Radiol 54:495–501
40. Smith DH, Meaney DF, Shull WH (2003) Diffuse axonal injury in head trauma. J Head Trauma Rehabil 18(4):307–316
41. Hafiz MZ, Saffari MH (2011) Characteristic differences in neuroimaging and physical findings between non-accidental and accidental traumatic brain injury in young children. A local experience in general hospital of Kuala Lumpur. Med J Malaysia 66(2):95–100
42. Moen KG, Skandsen T, Folvik M, Brezova V, Kvistad KA, Rydland J, Manley GT, Vik A (2012) A longitudinal MRI study of traumatic axonal injury in patients with moderate and severe traumatic brain injury. J Neurol Neurosurg Psychiatry 83(12):1193–1200
43. Scheid R, Preul C, Gruber O, Wiggins C, von Cramon DY (2003) Diffuse axonal injury associated with chronic traumatic brain injury: evidence from T2*-weighted gradient-echo imaging at 3 T. AJNR Am J Neuroradiol 24(6):1049–1056

Pediatric Thoracic Trauma

3

Stefania Ianniello, Vincenza Di Giacomo, Gavina Cuneo, Carmelo Rende, and Vittorio Miele

3.1 Introduction

Traumatic injury still remains the most common source of morbidity and mortality in children aged 1–14 years.

Thoracic trauma account for only 5–12 % of the admissions to trauma centers, but it may be associated with greater lethality. In fact, thoracic injuries account for approximately 14 % of blunt force traumatic deaths, second only to head injuries [1].

Between 60 and 80 % of chest injuries in younger children are the result of blunt trauma, with over half accounted for by impact with motor vehicles. In adolescents, however, penetrating trauma has a statistically more prominent role [2].

Injuries in the pediatric population tend to differ from those in adults because of anatomic, physiological, and epidemiologic differences. The greater flexibility of the thoracic cage results in fewer rib fractures and prevalence of pulmonary contusions. In addition, aortic tears and diaphragmatic lesions are very uncommon thanks to the increased mobility of the mediastinum in children.

On the other hand, the trachea is narrow, short, more compressible, and narrowest at the level of the cricoid cartilage; therefore, small changes in airway diameter may lead to rapid respiratory embarrassment [2, 3].

Every child with blunt thoracic trauma must be hospitalized and observed for immediate surgical interventions. Associated injury, especially head trauma, is the most important mortality factor. In a review of 137 children with blunt thoracic injury, Balci et al. [4] found that associated head, abdominal, and orthopedic injuries were present in 68.6–82 % of children with trauma and increased mortality and morbidity. Mortality for children with isolated chest trauma was 5 %, compared

S. Ianniello (✉) • V. Di Giacomo • G. Cuneo • C. Rende • V. Miele
Cardiovascular and Emergency Radiology Department, S. Camillo Hospital, C.ne Gianicolense, 87, Rome 00152, Italy
e-mail: stefianni66@gmail.com; vmiele@sirm.org

V. Miele, M. Trinci (eds.), *Imaging Trauma and Polytrauma in Pediatric Patients*,
DOI 10.1007/978-3-319-08524-1_3

with rates of 20 % for abdominal and chest trauma, 35 % for head and chest trauma, and 39 % for trauma to the head, chest, and abdomen.

3.2 Imaging Techniques

3.2.1 Chest Radiography

Screening chest radiographs are an important component of the evaluation of pediatric thoracic injury. They can be acquired rapidly and provide information about the locations of supportive lines and tubes and the presence of pulmonary lesions, pneumothorax, hemothorax, mediastinal lesions, etc. Because of the restrictions regarding immobilization of the cervical spine in trauma patients, anteroposterior (AP) chest radiograph is usually the most feasible initial study, but it is not as sensitive as the erect chest X-ray or computed tomography (CT) for detection of thoracic pathology.

Although CT may reveal clinically relevant thoracic lesions that were undetected by chest radiograph, AP chest radiograph still remains a cost-effective first-line tool in the imaging workup of pediatric thoracic trauma [5]. It has indisputable advantages such as widespread availability, relatively low cost, and easy acquisition.

3.2.2 Multidetector Computed Tomography

Recently, with the development and widespread availability of multidetector CT scanners, computed tomography has assumed a greater role in the noninvasive evaluation of chest trauma in children. Fast acquisition times, high spatial resolution and multiplanar reformation, and three-dimensional (3D) reconstructions make MDCT an ideal imaging method for evaluating chest injuries in the pediatric population when plain radiographs and ultrasound cannot provide all the necessary information for a correct diagnosis.

MDCT is more sensitive than chest radiography for a multitude of chest injuries such as rib fractures, pneumothorax, hemothorax, lung contusions and lacerations, diaphragmatic rupture, and aortic injuries. MDCT is not only accurate but also an "all-in-one" exam that allows a complete evaluation of the critically injured patient with a complete contiguous head-through-pelvis scan. Such total body scanning is advocated by many investigators for the adult population [6], but we should be more cautious before employing a similar protocol in the pediatric one. The finding of a study of Patel et al. suggests that chest CT should not be routinely used to evaluate all pediatric trauma patients. In children, aortic and other mediastinal injuries are uncommon if compared with the adults. According to this study, CT should be reserved for patients in whom the mechanism of injury or cardiovascular status is suggestive of spinal or vascular injury. They support the idea that abdominopelvic CT imaging that includes the lower chest might obviate the need for dedicated chest CT imaging when the suspicion for significant intrathoracic injury is low [7].

Table 3.1 Guidelines for tube current and kilovoltage

Weight	Tube current (mAs)	Kilovoltage (kVp)
<10	40	80
10–14	50	80
15–24	60	80
25–34	70	80
35–44	80	80
45–54	90	90
55–70	100–120	100–120

Pediatric CT examination should be performed at the lowest possible radiation dose level while also maintaining the highest image quality. The guidelines for tube current and kilovoltage are shown in Table 3.1 [8].

Routine pediatric thoracic CT protocols using intravenous iodinated contrast material are sufficient to diagnose the most clinically important chest traumatic lesions. Fast table speed (<1 s), thin detector collimation (<1 mm), and a 1–2 mm reconstruction interval are recommended to allow the creation of isotropic reformatted images as well as three-dimensional volume-rendered images of the aorta and the thoracic cage. CT angiography (either with or without electrocardiogram gating) is the preferable imaging study when there is a high suspicion of aortic pathology [1, 8].

3.2.3 Chest Ultrasound

Emerging indications of ultrasound include the evaluation of pneumothoraces, costochondral and rib fractures, and even pulmonary contusions.

In patients with major trauma, the initial US examination is generally performed with a FAST (focused assessment with sonography in trauma) protocol that is effective in depicting intraperitoneal collections of free fluid that are an indirect sign of solid organ injury and require urgent surgical exploration. After the initial FAST survey, the US examination may be rapidly extended to the thorax to rule out hemothorax and pneumothorax or to guide interventional procedures such as endotracheal intubation. This "extended to thorax" examination is called extended FAST (e-FAST).

In the trauma setting, the FAST examination is usually performed in hypotensive and hemodynamically unstable patients because it helps determine whether immediate surgery is needed before the patient undergoes a CT evaluation; in fact, if an intra-abdominal bleeding is present, the probability of death increases by about 1 % for every 3 min that elapses before surgical exploration [9].

In a meta-analysis by Ding et al. comparing the use of anteroposterior chest radiography with transthoracic ultrasonography for the diagnosis of pneumothorax, pooled sensitivity and specificity were 88 and 99 %, respectively, for ultrasonography and 52 and 100 %, respectively, for CR [10].

As with sonography elsewhere in the body, the appropriate transducers and frequencies vary with the size of the patient and the structure examined. Neonates and small infants are easily examined with high-frequency linear transducers, whereas older children require lower-frequency transducers. Basic B-mode real-time is generally all that is required for chest US. The use of M-mode imaging could be helpful in the evaluation of pneumothorax [11].

Current trends in pediatric imaging support the increased use of ultrasound to decrease radiation exposure. Unfortunately, at this time, ultrasound cannot replace other imaging modalities in the setting of acute pediatric thoracic trauma because of a variety of inherent limitations and its operator dependence. We believe that this imaging method could answer to specific clinical questions during the acute resuscitation period.

3.2.4 Other Imaging Modalities

Catheter-based angiography of the thoracic aorta is performed far less frequently than in the past, as CT angiography has been accepted as an accurate diagnostic tool for the diagnosis of acute aortic injury. It should be used only in cases of equivocal CT findings [12].

Magnetic resonance imaging (MRI) carries major drawbacks in the acute emergency setting such as longer acquisition times, inability to closely observe the patient within the MRI scanner, and prohibition to introduce ferromagnetic devices. For this reason, MRI is rarely indicated in children after thoracic trauma. MRI is commonly indicated in the evaluation of spinal cord lesions in cases of abnormality of the neurologic examination or unexplained severe spinal pain after thoracic trauma [2].

3.3 Radiation Dose Consideration in Pediatric Examinations

A single chest radiograph exposes a patient to a dose of 0.02 millisievert (mSv), whereas a CT of the chest exposes the patient to roughly 8 mSv of ionizing radiation [13].

A retrospective study from Pearce et al. suggests that radiation doses of 50–60 mGy (2–3 head CTs) in children could triple their risk of brain tumors [14].

Children are more prone to radiation-induced cancers and have a longer expected life span than adults. Although there are multiple imaging modalities in the trauma specialist's arsenal, the use of CT has increased exponentially also in children. Despite this trend, chest radiograph remains an acceptable screening tool to analyze which patients may require CT evaluation.

The ALARA (as low as reasonably achievable) principle aims to balance appropriate use and low-dose imaging with imaging quality; it refers to a campaign to reduce the amount of ionizing radiation exposure by using specialized pediatric protocols and using alternate modalities when possible [13].

Blunt thoracic trauma can result in life-threatening emergencies. CT will frequently be necessary for its high specificity and sensitivity in the detection of thoracic trauma lesions. The concept of ALARA should never be used to withhold a gold standard diagnostic test from a sick child. Chest CT scanning is particularly important in children with chest trauma when hemodynamic instability or respiratory failure requiring intubation develops or when there is persistent drainage of blood or air from chest tubes or a progressive pneumomediastinum.

Alternative imaging modalities to CT, such as MRI and US, should be considered to answer specific clinical questions during the observation period.

3.4 Lung Parenchymal Injuries

3.4.1 Contusion

A major difference between adults and children is the compliance of the chest wall, due to greater elasticity of the ribs. This allows greater deformation of the chest before the ribs fracture. Thus, major internal injuries may occur without any external chest injury.

Pulmonary contusions are the most common finding in pediatric patients after a blunt chest trauma. This condition is the result of the direct impact of adjacent bony structures such as ribs and spine on the lung parenchyma, leading to focal hemorrhage, edema, and/or alveolar collapse.

Lung contusions become apparent on chest radiographs with some delay of up to 6 h [3, 15].

They are more reliably demonstrated on CT scans as peripherally located ground-glass or consolidative airspace opacities, not always associated to rib fractures; they typically exhibit a thin zone of surrounding subpleural lucency. Most contusions resolve in 2–7 days.

The differential diagnosis includes atelectasis and aspiration pneumonia that are typically located in the dependent portions of the lung and have a segmental distribution.

While in the adults large pulmonary contusions (involving at least 20 % of the lung parenchyma) can lead to acute respiratory distress syndrome, increased need of mechanical ventilation, and increased mortality, in children these injuries do not appear to have the same degree of morbidity [1].

In recent studies, US has been shown in adults to be more sensitive than chest radiography for the diagnosis of pulmonary contusion, with sensitivity and specificity rates of >90 % [16]. Also in children, the relatively high radiation dose associated with CT may be avoided by the use of US (Fig. 3.1).

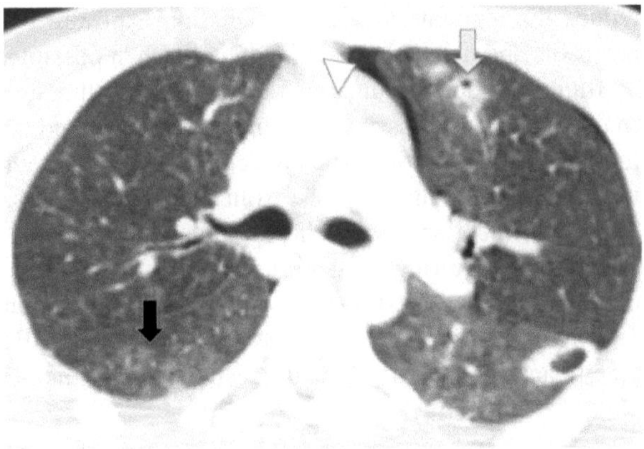

Fig. 3.1 A 14-year-old male with blunt chest trauma. Axial CT image demonstrates left-sided pulmonary laceration (*white arrow*), left-sided pneumothorax (*white arrowhead*), and right lower lobe contusions (*black arrow*)

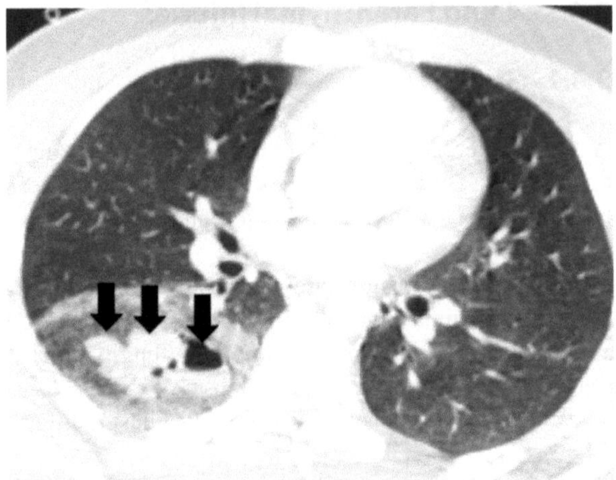

Fig. 3.2 A 13-year-old male with blunt chest trauma. Axial CT image demonstrates right-sided round or oval collections of air and/or blood suggestive of hemato-pneumatocele (*arrows*). Note that they are central and surrounded by lung contusions

3.4.2 Pneumatocele

Pneumatoceles are caused by the rupture of the most distal airways resulting from abnormal forces applied to the compliant pediatric chest. They appear as round or oval collections of air and/or blood (hemato-pneumatocele), are usually central and surrounded by lung contusions, and vary in size from a few millimeters to several centimeters [1] (Figs. 3.2, 3.3, and 3.4).

3.4.3 Laceration

Pulmonary lacerations are derived from penetrating injuries, rib fractures, or compressive shear on the lung at the time of the blunt injury and consist of a

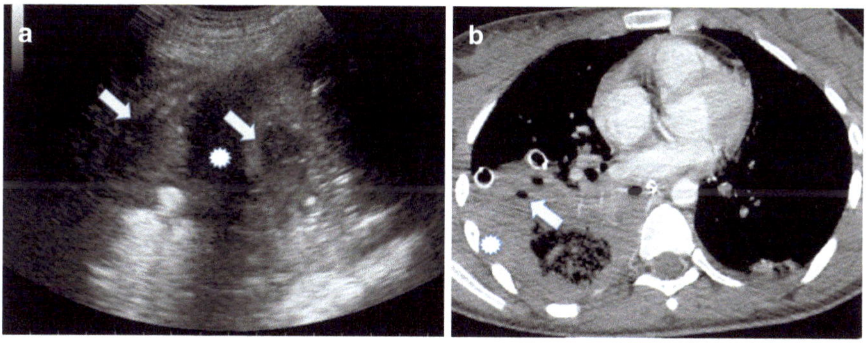

Fig. 3.3 A 12-year-old male with blunt chest trauma. Ultrasonographic scan (**a**) of the base of the right lung demonstrates multiple fluid collections (*arrows* in **a**) and pleural effusion (*asterisk*). Axial CT image (**b**) demonstrates right-sided round or oval collections of air and/or blood suggestive of hemato-pneumatocele (*arrows* in **b**) and pleural effusion (*asterisk*). Note the presence of hemothorax

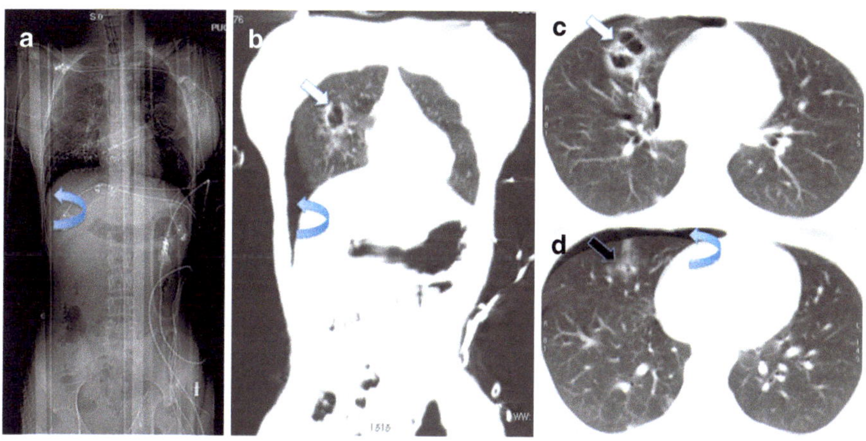

Fig. 3.4 A 14-year-old male with blunt chest trauma. CT scanogram (**a**) shows the *deep sulcus sign* (*curved arrow* in **a**). Coronal reformatted multidetector-row CT image (**b**) and axial multidetector-row CT images (**c** and **d**) show the presence of pneumothorax (*curved arrow* in **b** and **d**) and right-sided pneumatoceles (*white arrow* in **b** and **c**). A small contusion is also present (*black arrow* in **d**)

disruption of the lung parenchyma. On CT, they appear as linear areas of lucency and are more easily demonstrated on reformatted images (Fig. 3.5).

Large lacerations involving the pleural surface may cause the development of a bronchopleural fistula.

Usually these lesions resolve more slowly than contusions, and especially in the pediatric patients, they may leave behind a persistent cavity called "post-traumatic pseudocyst" [1–3, 15].

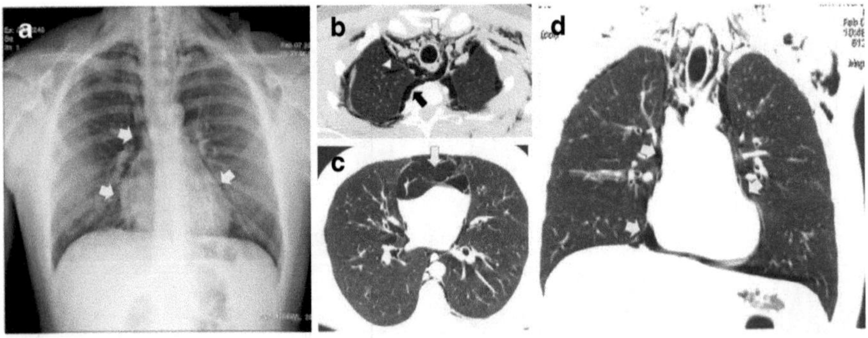

Fig. 3.5 A 14-year-old male with blunt chest trauma. On chest radiograph, (**a**) note the presence of pneumomediastinum (*white arrow*) and subcutaneous emphysema (*red arrow*). Axial CT images (**b** and **c**) and coronal reformatted CT image (**d**) demonstrate the presence of a linear area of lucency in the right upper lobe consistent with parenchymal laceration (*white arrowhead* in **b**), extensive pneumomediastinum (*white arrow* in **b–d**), right-sided pneumothorax (*black arrow* in **b**), and subcutaneous emphysema

3.5 Pleural Space Abnormalities

3.5.1 Pneumothorax

Traumatic pneumothorax occurs via blunt or penetrating mechanism. Usually, air enters the pleural space from pulmonary, chest wall, esophageal, or tracheobronchial tree injuries. Rib fractures may not be present in children.

The most concerning adverse outcome of traumatic pneumothorax is progression to a tension pneumothorax. This occurs when the air flows into the pleural cavity without a means of escape, resulting in mediastinal shift, reduced venous blood return to the heart, and a rapid decline in cardiac output. The typical indicators that a pneumothorax is under tension are the mediastinal shift to the contralateral side, depression of the ipsilateral diaphragm, and rapid expansion on serial radiographs.

Pneumothorax occurs in one-third of pediatric thoracic traumas, with the majority of these having associated intrathoracic and extrathoracic injuries and only one-third occurring in isolation. Vital signs and symptomatology depend on the size of the pneumothorax. Patients may present in moderate to severe distress, and tachycardia, hypotension, and oxygen desaturation are also seen [17].

In patients presenting with multiple trauma, an upright chest radiograph cannot be performed. Supine anteroposterior chest radiograph is unreliable at detecting pneumothorax, with a sensitivity of 36–48 % in some studies. Subtle findings include a sharply defined diaphragm or an inferior lung border or cardiac border. Some patients may exhibit the *deep sulcus sign*, which represents lucency of the lateral costophrenic angle extending toward the hypochondrium and giving the deepened lateral costophrenic angle a very sharp appearance [18, 19].

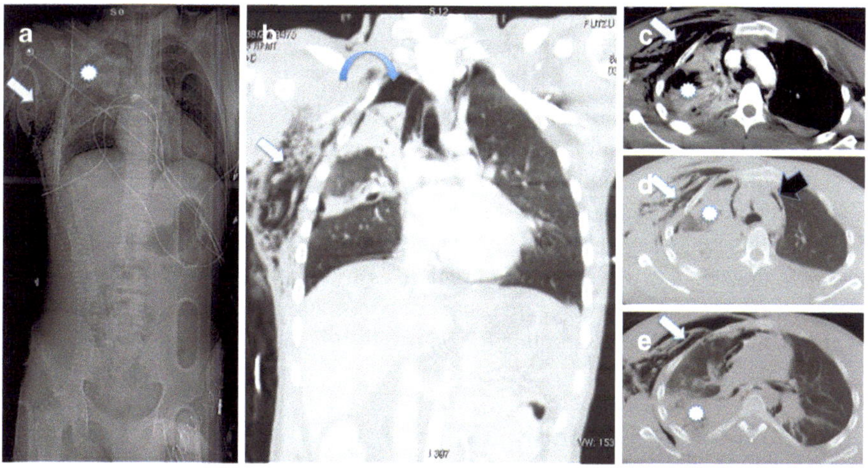

Fig. 3.6 A 15-year-old male with blunt chest trauma. CT scanogram (**a**), coronal reformatted CT image (**b**), and axial CT images (**c–e**) demonstrate the presence of large contusions (*asterisk* in **a**, **c–e**), right-sided pneumothorax (*curved arrow* in **b**), subcutaneous emphysema (*white arrow* in **a–e**), and pneumomediastinum (*black arrow* in **d**)

With the introduction and increased availability of multidetector CT scanners, chest CT has become the reference standard examination in the diagnosis of traumatic pneumothorax.

As expected, CT is more sensitive for small pneumothoraces than chest radiography [20]. Most of this *occult pneumothoraces* (pneumothoraces not seen on chest radiography) remain clinically silent. However, if the patient undergoes positive-pressure ventilation for any cause, they may enlarge causing cardiorespiratory compromise.

Ultrasound has become more readily available at the bedside in the trauma setting. Several authors have investigated the accuracy of US for the detection of pneumothorax in adult trauma patients and in those who have sustained interventional procedures such as lung biopsy [21]. In a study of Soldati et al., the sensitivity and specificity of chest US in detecting PNX were 92 and 99.4 %, respectively, if compared to CT as the reference standard [22].

In a retrospective study of 368 adult patients with major chest trauma, we found an accuracy of 97.2 % for chest ultrasound in the diagnosis of pneumothorax compared with MDCT and thoracostomy tube placement [23] (Figs. 3.4, 3.5, and 3.6).

We believe that ultrasound will play a major role in the evaluation of traumatic pneumothorax in the near future, in children.

3.5.2 Hemothorax, Chylothorax, and Cholothorax

Hemothorax is the result of arterial or venous bleeding into the pleural cavity and occurs in about 13 % of pediatric trauma patients. The vascular injury may be the result of tearing from rapid deceleration or laceration from an adjacent rib fracture. On supine chest radiography, hemothorax manifests as a veillike increased density over the involved hemithorax, often associated to ipsilateral rib fractures. At CT, hemothorax appears as a high-attenuation pleural fluid (between 50 and 80 HU); active contrast extravasation into the pleural space is rarely seen by CT in children.

Once diagnosed, blood should be promptly evacuated to avoid the development of empyema and fibrothorax.

Chylothorax is a collection of lymphatic fluid within the pleural space due to thoracic duct injury, while cholothorax derives from extravasation of bile into the thoracic cavity. They are very rare causes of post-traumatic pleural space fluid collections and require fluid sampling to confirm the diagnosis [1, 2, 18].

3.6 Mediastinal Abnormalities

3.6.1 Pneumomediastinum

Pneumomediastinum (free air within the mediastinum) is observed in 5–10 % of all patients with blunt thoracic trauma.

It may be caused by direct penetrating injury, tracheobronchial or esophageal rupture, and in the absence of demonstrable visceral injury, it has also been attributed to the so-called Macklin effect. This phenomenon consists of a sudden rise in intra-alveolar pressure resulting in alveolar rupture, interstitial emphysema, and ultimately pneumomediastinum.

Free mediastinal air does not always indicate thoracic injury; extrathoracic causes of gas in the mediastinum include head and neck trauma as well as subdiaphragmatic pathology.

At chest radiography, pneumomediastinum can manifest as mediastinal linear lucencies, as the "continuous diaphragm" sign, caused by air outlining the superior diaphragmatic surface, or as the "spinnaker sail" sign, resulting from mediastinal air elevating the thymic lobes.

CT is more reliable than chest radiograph in demonstrating even small amount of air in the mediastinum and differentiating pneumomediastinum from a pneumothorax [1, 24] (Fig. 3.5).

3.6.2 Esophageal Injury

Rupture of the esophagus is rarely seen after chest trauma in children (occurring in <0.1 %).

When present, however, this condition manifests with pneumomediastinum and a left-sided pleural effusion. A combined tracheal and esophageal injury may lead to the development of a traumatic tracheoesophageal fistula (0.001 % of all thoracic trauma patients). The diagnosis requires a contrast esophagogram, chest CT, or bronchoscopy.

Esophageal injuries typically require a surgical treatment [24].

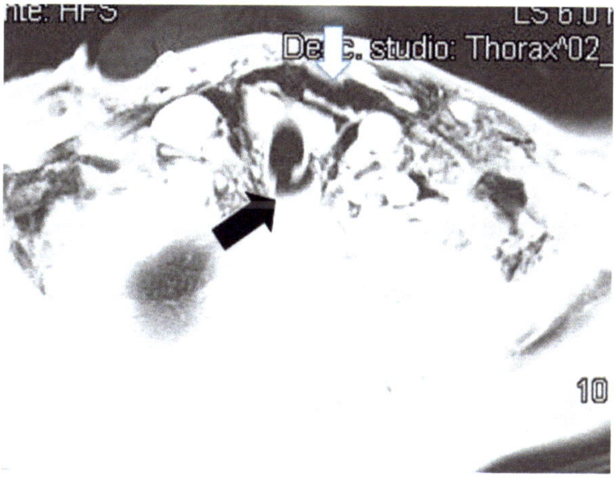

Fig. 3.7 A 15-year-old male with blunt chest trauma. Axial multidetector-row CT image shows focal disruption of the posterior aspect of the proximal trachea (*black arrow*). Pneumomediastinum (*white arrow*) and subcutaneous emphysema are also present

3.6.3 Tracheobronchial Injury

Tracheobronchial injuries, related to either penetrating or blunt chest trauma, are fortunately rare in children, accounting for <1 % of pediatric patients with thoracic trauma. In blunt trauma, the injury may result either from compression of the sternum against the spine or from a sudden increase in intrathoracic pressure against a closed glottis.

Although the overall incidence is low, traumatic tracheobronchial lesions are associated with a mortality rate of up to 30 %, mainly due to delayed diagnosis. The most common locations are the distal trachea, just above the carina, and proximal bronchi, especially the right main bronchus. Rib fractures are seen in 25 % of cases of tracheobronchial rupture, especially those involving the anterior ends of the first three ribs.

Typically, these patients exhibit persistent pneumothorax and/or pneumomediastinum, even in the presence of a well-functioning chest tube and/or mediastinal tube. Another common finding is subcutaneous emphysema.

In cases of complete transection or rupture of the main bronchus, the "fallen lung sign" may be visible on chest radiographs, which represents the collapsed lung located in a dependent position, hanging on the hilum only by its vascular attachments.

Many airway injuries may be diagnosed by rigid or flexible bronchoscopy. Also MDCT with thin-section axial and 2D/3D reconstructions can help accurately diagnose tracheobronchial injuries in the pediatric population [15, 18, 24, 25].

Due to their high lethality, most of these lesions require prompt diagnosis and surgical treatment; distal bronchial injuries are generally managed by anatomic pulmonary resection, whereas lesions of the proximal tracheobronchial tree are repaired surgically.

The possible late sequelae are airway stenosis, atelectasis, and pneumonia [2] (Fig. 3.7).

3.6.4 Aortic Injury

Aortic laceration is very rare, occurring in less than 0.1 % of children presenting with blunt thoracic trauma. However, the overall mortality is approximately 40 %, with the majority of deaths occurring at the time of injury. Children who sustain a traumatic thoracic aortic injury will also have important injuries to other organs (lung contusions in 100 %).

The most common site of aortic tear is the isthmus, distal to the left subclavian artery and at the level of the ligamentum arteriosum. This is the site where the relatively mobile aortic arch becomes fixed at the descending aorta and, therefore, more prone to injury from traumatic shearing forces. The mechanism of aortic injury is believed to be the ligamentum arteriosum tethering the aorta at the moment of the shearing trauma, leading to a tear in the intima and media. The adventitia is the only layer holding the aorta together, accounting for the instability of this pseudoaneurysm and a high mortality (80–85 %).

Another sign of traumatic aortic injury is the presence of a mediastinal hematoma. Despite its limitations, AP chest radiograph obtained in the trauma room may be the first screening for this condition, which carries a great lethality.

The common diagnostic criteria published in the adult literature (mediastinal width greater than 8 cm, mediastinum-to-chest ratio greater than 0.25) lack proven accuracy for traumatic aortic injury in children.

Of greater value are other imaging findings on chest radiograph, such as obliterated contour of the aortic arch, blurring of the aortopulmonary window, deviation of trachea and nasogastric tube to the right, downward depression of the left mainstem bronchus, widening of the paravertebral and paratracheal stripes, and a left apical pleural cap. Unfortunately, these signs are not sufficiently specific, so that the positive predictive value for detecting aortic injury with chest radiograph is low (5–20 %). On the contrary, a normal chest radiograph has a high predictive value to rule out aortic rupture (96 %).

The most common finding of aortic injury demonstrated with MDCT is a pseudoaneurysm located on the anterior aspect of the proximal descending aorta; this pseudoaneurysm is not to be confused with the ductus diverticulum ("ductus bump"), a remnant of the ductus arteriosus that can normally be found in this location.

Other signs are a periaortic hematoma, intimal flaps, wall irregularities, abrupt caliber changes, occlusion of major branch vessels, luminal clots, and active contrast extravasation [2, 15, 18, 24].

Multidetector-row CT angiography has become accepted as an accurate diagnostic test for acute aortic injury. In a study by Dyer et al., CT had 100 % sensitivity and 100 % negative predictive value for the detection of traumatic aortic injury [26] (Figs. 3.8, 3.9, 3.10, 3.11, 3.12, 3.13, and 3.14).

3.6.5 Cardiac and Pericardial Injury

Cardiac injury is a rare event in the setting of pediatric thoracic trauma and occurs more frequently with penetrating compared with blunt chest trauma. Myocardial

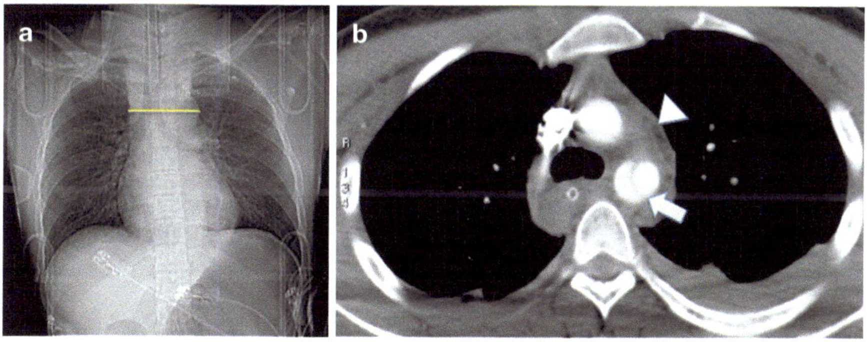

Fig. 3.8 A 14-year-old male with blunt chest trauma. CT scanogram (**a**) shows an abnormally widened mediastinum. Axial multidetector-row CT image at the level of the aortic isthmus (**b**) shows a periaortic hematoma (*arrowhead*) and the intimal flap (*arrow*) consistent with an aortic isthmic tear

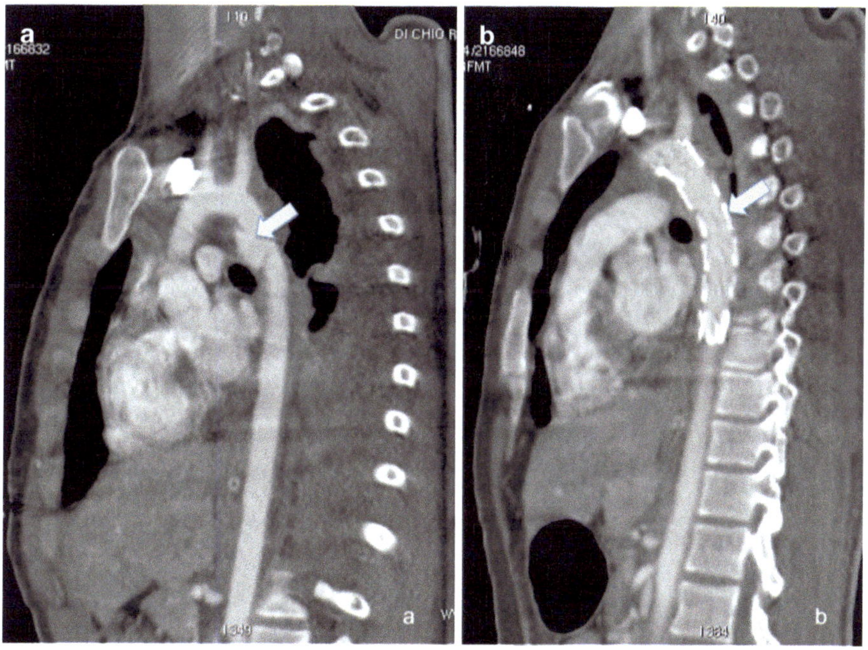

Fig. 3.9 Same case of Fig. 3.5. Sagittal reformatted multidetector-row CT image (**a**) shows aortic pseudoaneurysm at the aortic isthmus (*arrow* in **a**). The patient underwent endovascular treatment; sagittal reformatted multidetector-row CT image (**b**) shows successful placement of a stent graft (*arrow* in **b**)

contusions represent more than 95 % of cardiac injuries due to blunt trauma, with ventricular laceration or rupture and valvular disruption occurring much less commonly.

Myocardial contusions are typically occult; they can be suspected on the basis of abnormal electrocardiographic findings or elevation of cardiac enzymes. Pneumopericardium appears as abnormal lucency within the pericardial space at

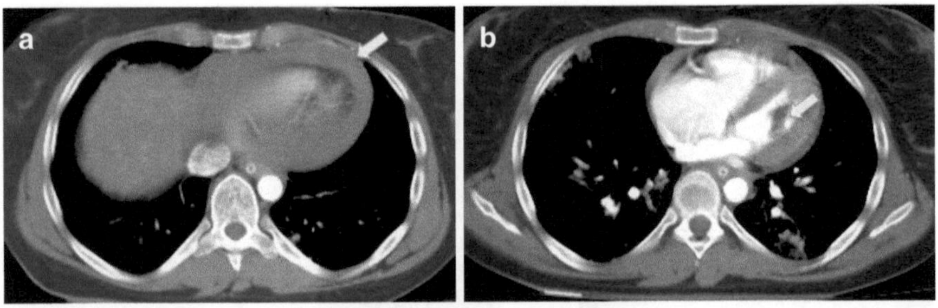

Fig. 3.10 A 13-year-old male with penetrating chest trauma. Axial CT scan shows a traumatic hemopericardium (*arrow* in **a**) and a thrombus (*arrow* in **b**) within the left ventricular cavity. The diagnosis of blunt cardiac injury was confirmed on the basis of abnormal electrocardiographic findings, elevated cardiac enzyme levels, and echocardiographic findings

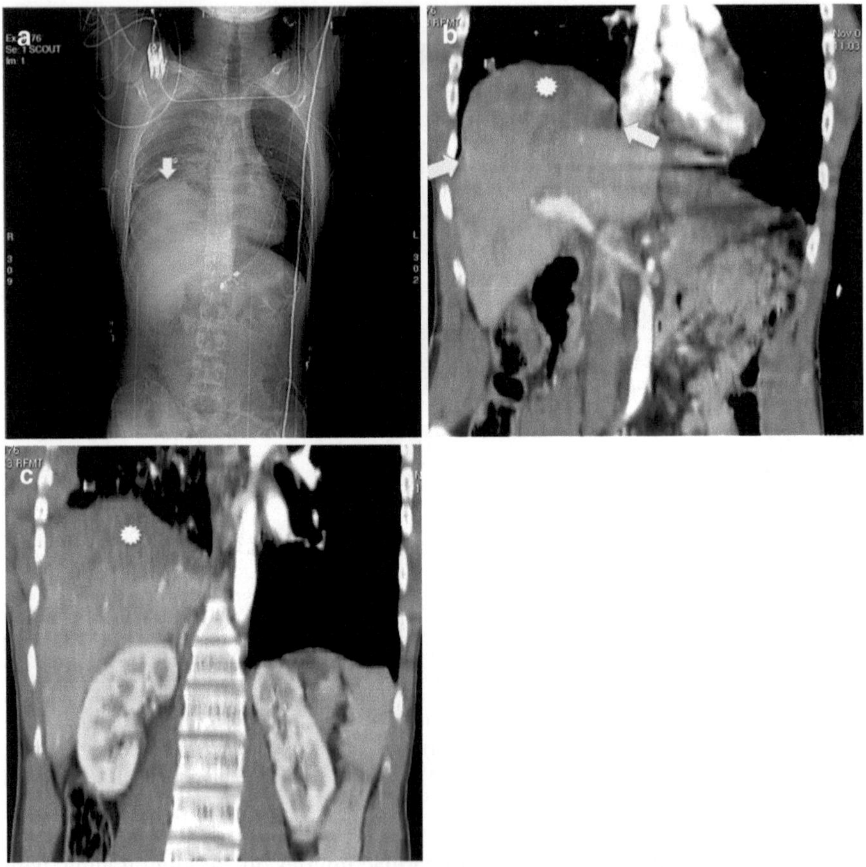

Fig. 3.11 A 15-year-old male with blunt chest trauma. CT scanogram (**a**) shows elevation of the right hemidiaphragm (*arrow*). Coronal reformatted multidetector-row CT images (**b, c**) show focal disruption of the right hemidiaphragm with herniation and constriction of the liver through the edges of the diaphragmatic tear (*rim* sign) (*arrow* in **b**). Note also the massive contusion of the hepatic dome (*asterisks* in **b, c**)

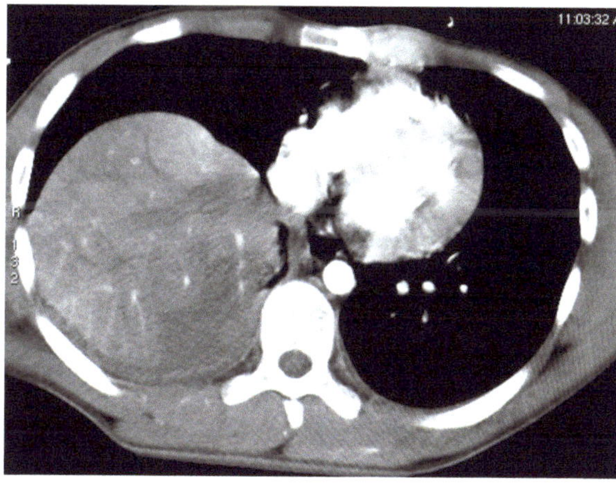

Fig. 3.12 Same case of Fig. 3.8. Axial multidetector-row CT image shows intrathoracic herniation of the liver. In the hepatic dome, multiple contusions and lacerations are present

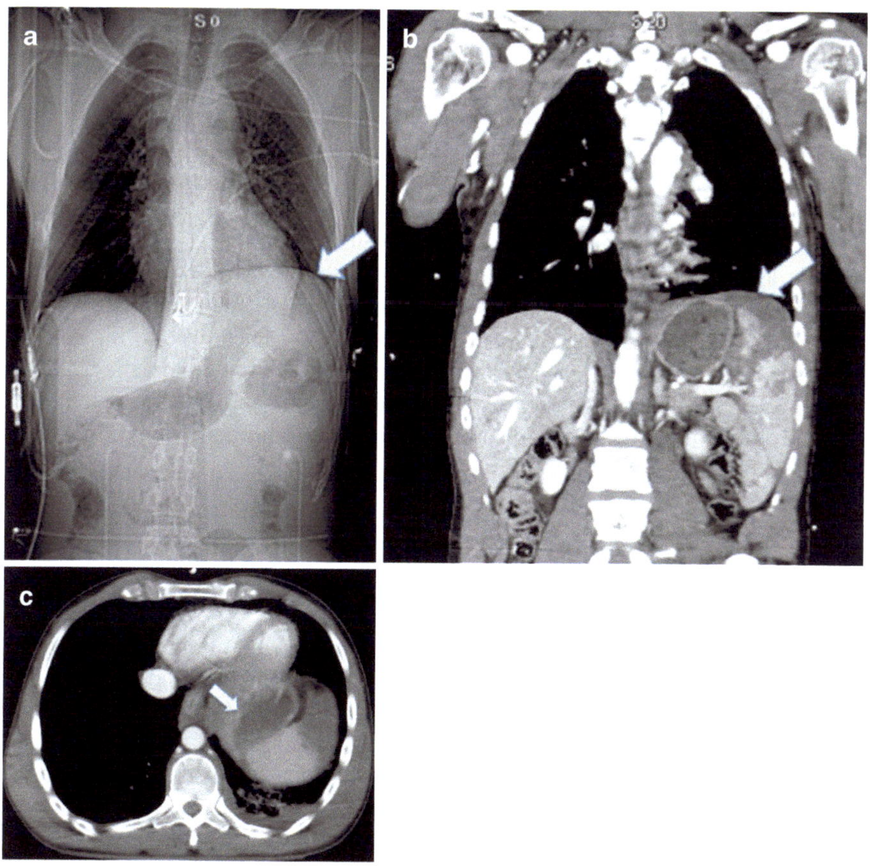

Fig. 3.13 A 14-year-old male with blunt chest trauma. CT scanogram (**a**) and coronal reformatted multidetector-row CT image (**b**) show elevation of the left hemidiaphragm (*arrow* in **a**, **b**). Axial CT image (**c**) shows herniation of the stomach and the spleen (*arrow* in **c**) through the edges of the diaphragmatic tear. A severe splenic trauma is also present

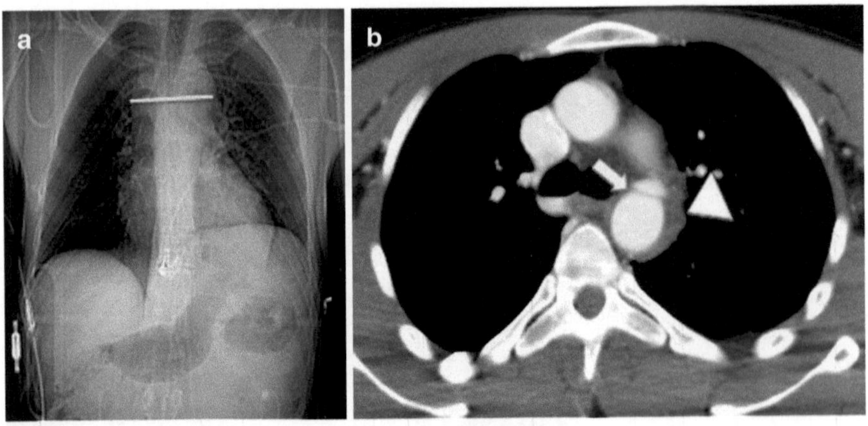

Fig. 3.14 Same case of Fig. 3.10. CT scanogram (**a**) shows an abnormally widened mediastinum. Axial multidetector-row CT image at the level of the aortic isthmus (**b**) shows a periaortic hematoma (*arrowhead*) and the intimal flap (*arrow*). These findings suggest an aortic isthmic tear

both radiography and CT. Hemopericardium causes an abnormal enlargement of the pericardial silhouette at radiography and accumulation of high-attenuation fluid within the pericardial space at CT.

Both pneumopericardium and hemopericardium can result in cardiac tamponade and require emergent surgical decompression.

Fortunately, most cardiac injuries resolve without sequelae. Less than 5 % of patients develop long-term complications, such as valvular dysfunction [1, 15, 18, 24].

"Commotio cordis" is a unique phenomenon in pediatric thoracic trauma, causing sudden death after discrete blunt chest trauma. It is characterized by the absence of cardiac contusion, coronary arterial abnormalities, structural anomalies, or conduction system pathology. Currently, it is thought that an abrupt strike to the chest in some children will result in a disorganized rhythm followed by rapid cardiovascular collapse [2] (Fig. 3.10).

3.7 Diaphragmatic Injury

The incidence of diaphragmatic rupture following major chest trauma in children is 1–5 %, usually as a consequence of a motor-vehicle accident. Left-sided injuries are more common than the right ones (reported rates of 70–80 % on the left side, 15–24 % on the right side, and 5–8 % bilaterally), and the site of the rupture is usually posterolateral. The explanation for the side discrepancy was believed to be the protective effect of the liver, but more recently, this long-held belief has been questioned with evidence that the incidence of right-sided diaphragmatic rupture may be underestimated.

As a consequence of a diaphragmatic tear, intra-abdominal viscera may herniate into the thoracic cavity with risk of strangulation and lung compression. On the left side, the most commonly herniated organs are the bowel (stomach, small bowel, and colon) and spleen, while on the right side, the liver is most commonly involved.

The AP chest radiograph is not very sensitive in the diagnosis of diaphragmatic rupture usually due to the presence of associated injuries, such as atelectasis, pulmonary contusions, and pleural effusions. Furthermore, visceral herniation may not occur until positive-pressure ventilation has been withdrawn resulting in a delayed diagnosis.

Radiographic findings may include apparent elevation of a hemidiaphragm, intrathoracic gas-filled stomach or bowel loops, and a nasogastric tube tip located within the chest.

MDCT with multiplanar reconstructions allows to delineate the exact site of the diaphragmatic tear, establish which abdominal viscera have herniated into the thorax, and identify other sites of injury.

Left-sided injuries are more easily diagnosed than right-sided injuries on CT images, with accuracy rates of 88 and 70 %, respectively.

The most sensitive imaging finding of a diaphragmatic rupture is the interruption of a hemidiaphragm, a subtle finding that indicates the need of a surgical repair to prevent future visceral or mesenteric fat herniation. The *hourglass* or *collar* sign refers to the waist-like constriction of partially herniated viscera by the edges of a small diaphragmatic tear. The *rim* sign is the term used for the same phenomenon in the liver. Other diagnostic criteria of diaphragmatic rupture are the *curled* diaphragm sign, a focal thickening of the diaphragm, and the *dependent viscera* sign referring to herniated viscera apposing the posterior chest wall without interposition of the lung parenchyma or diaphragm.

Diaphragmatic ruptures may be initially overlooked and diagnosed only at a later stage when the patient re-presents with complications such as visceral herniation and/or strangulation [15, 18] (Figs. 3.11, 3.12, and 3.13).

3.8 Chest Wall Injuries

3.8.1 Rib Fractures

The pediatric chest wall has greater flexibility when compared to adults as a result of increased ligamentous laxity and less rib mineralization. Pediatric ribs typically bend instead of breaking when compressed, so that more of the trauma energy is dissipated to the thoracic content. Consequently, rib fractures occur less frequently than in adults, and major intrathoracic pathology may occur even in the absence of rib fractures [3].

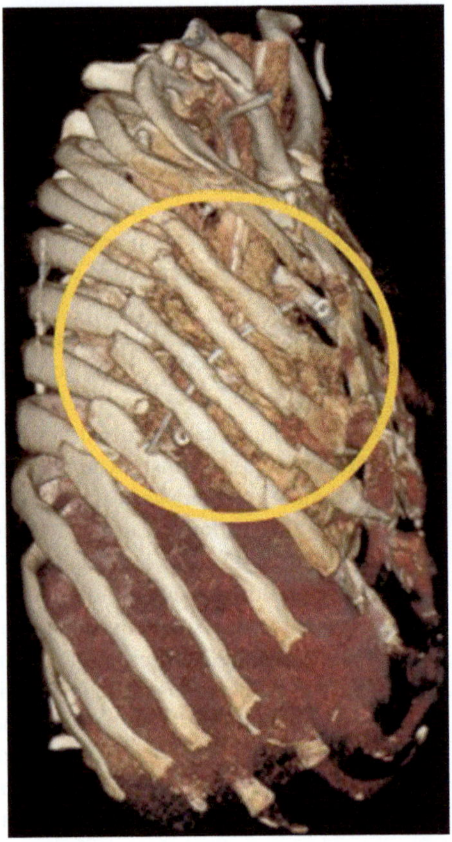

Fig. 3.15 A 16-year-old boy with blunt chest trauma. Volume-rendered CT image of a "flail chest" (*circle*)

In children, rib fractures are commonly posterior in location while in the adults are lateral.

Multiple rib fractures occur more commonly than a single isolated fracture and are associated with a greater incidence of multiorgan trauma, 70 % versus 12 %.

Fractures of the upper ribs, usually caused by high-energy trauma, are often combined with severe either vascular or esophago-tracheobronchial injuries; lower rib fractures are often combined with laceration of the upper abdominal organs.

When nondisplaced, acute rib fractures are typically very difficult to diagnose on an AP chest radiograph and are missed more than 50 % of the time. Although CT is more sensitive, the identification of such lesions does not significantly impact patient management.

A "flail chest" is the result of parallel double fractures of two or more adjacent ribs with subsequent loss of the bony continuity of the thoracic cavity. This is fortunately a rare injury, with an incidence of just 1 %. The result is a paradoxical chest wall movement in the flail segment leading to respiratory distress (Fig. 3.15) [15, 18, 24].

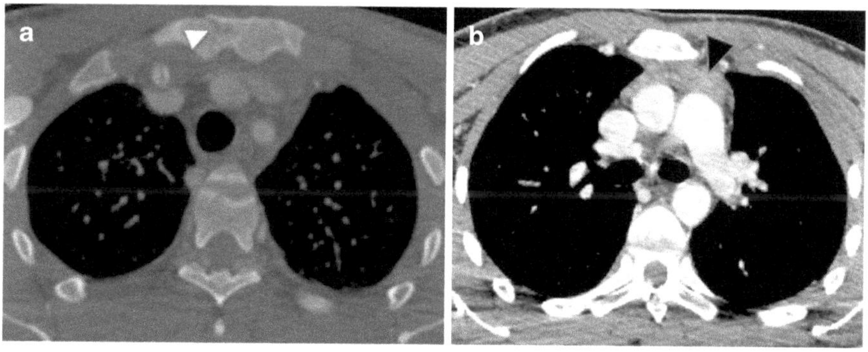

Fig. 3.16 Axial multidetector-row CT images of a sternal fracture after a road accident in a 13-year-old girl. The fracture is located at the level of the manubrium (*arrowhead* in **a**) and is associated to a mediastinal hematoma (*arrowhead* in **b**)

3.8.2 Sternal Fractures

Sternal fractures and posterior sternoclavicular dislocations typically occur in the setting of high-impact trauma and represent a diagnostic dilemma because they are generally indicative of more serious underlying problems, such as vascular, tracheal, and even cardiac injuries.

Sternal fractures are seen with an increasing frequency in road accidents, especially after the introduction of seat belt legislation. Such fractures are usually transverse and are localized most commonly to the midbody, followed by the manubrium (Fig. 3.16) [1].

3.8.3 Thoracic Spine Injuries

Thoracic spine injuries may occur in a variety of settings. Axial loading, such as that experienced in football or falls, may result in compression injuries. Translational deceleration may result in spinal cord or ligamentous injury from hyperflexion or hyperextension.

Most injuries are motor-vehicle related (50 %); also, falls account for a high percentage (24 %).

CT is more sensitive than radiography in the detection of spine fractures. MRI is indicated to evaluate for spinal cord injury in the setting of spinal canal narrowing due to fracture fragment retropulsion.

Vertebral body compression fractures are typically the consequence of hyperflexion. This type of fracture is the most common type of thoracic spine fracture and is best visualized on lateral radiographs or sagittal reformatted CT images.

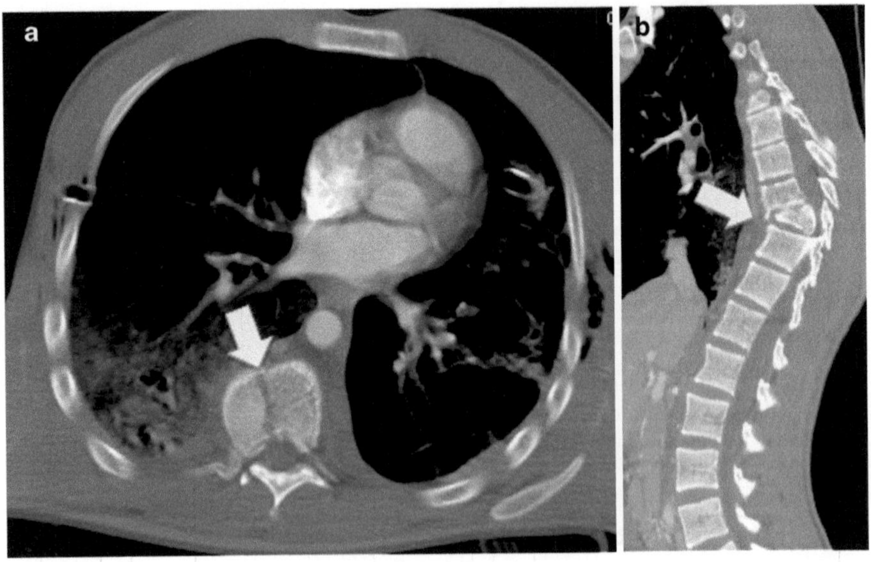

Fig. 3.17 Severe fracture-dislocation in the midthoracic spine in a 14-year-old boy who has sustained major injury in a motor-vehicle accident. Axial (**a**) and sagittal (**b**) images of multidetector-row CT show unstable fracture (*arrows* in **a**, **b**) with focal kyphosis and impingement of the spinal canal by bone fragments. Also, note right lung contusion and bilateral pleural fluid

A burst fracture, usually due to axial loading of the spine, is characterized by loss of vertebral body height, fracture lines involving both the anterior and posterior vertebral body cortices, and fracture fragment retropulsion into the spinal canal. These fractures are best diagnosed on axial and sagittal CT reformatted images.

Chance (or seat belt) fractures are caused by hyperflexion-distraction trauma that can occur during a motor-vehicle accident in which the patient was restrained using only a lap belt and no shoulder restraint. These fractures, usually observed in the lower thoracic or upper lumbar spine, consist of a horizontal fracture line through the posterior aspect of the vertebral body. These lesions may be often associated in children to anterior abdominal wall, bowel, mesentery, and solid organ injuries. Chance fractures are generally very conspicuous on sagittal and coronal CT reformatted images.

Finally, especially in younger children, spinal cord injury (hemorrhage, transection, or central cord syndrome) may occur without disruption of the bony anatomy due to the excessive mobility of the pediatric spine [1, 18, 24].

MRI is the most useful diagnostic tool in the setting of spinal cord injury without radiologic abnormality [2] (Figs. 3.17 and 3.18).

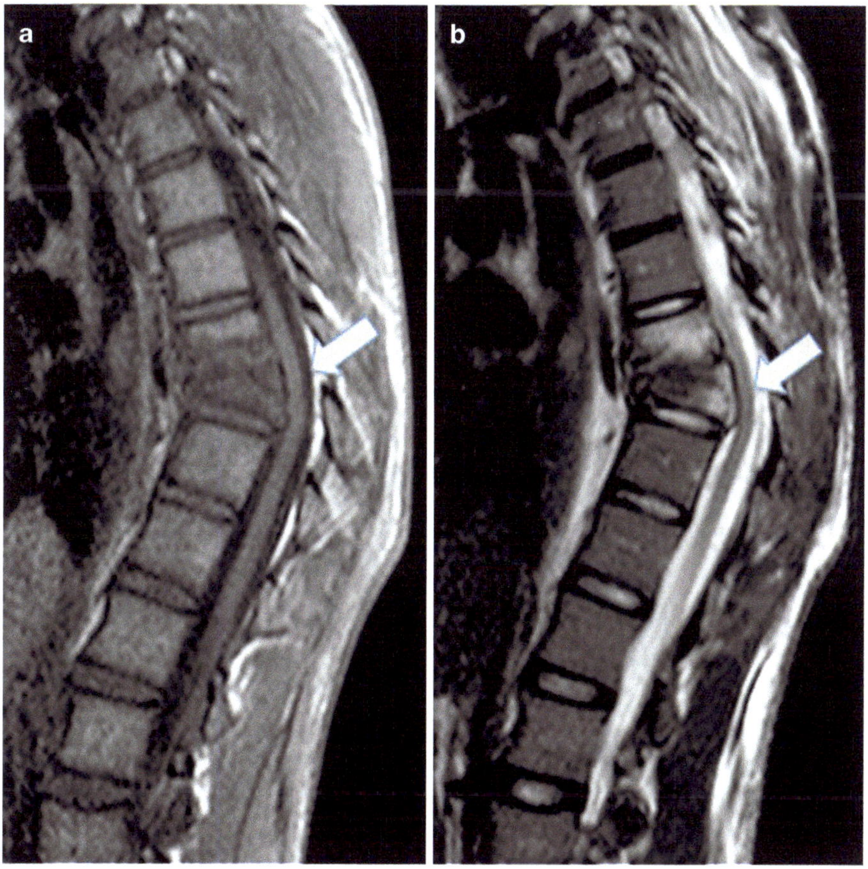

Fig. 3.18 Same case of Fig. 3.14. MRI is indicated to evaluate for spinal cord injury in the setting of spinal canal narrowing due to fracture fragment retropulsion. Sagittal T1-weighted (**a**) and T2-weighted (**b**) MR images show unstable fracture with focal kyphosis. Spinal cord exhibits normal signal intensity (*arrows* in **a**, **b**)

References

1. Hammer MR, Dillman JR, Chong ST, Strouse PJ (2012) Imaging of pediatric thoracic trauma. Semin Roentgenol 47(2):135–146
2. Bliss D, Silen M (2002) Pediatric thoracic trauma. Crit Care Med 30(11 suppl):S409–S415
3. Bisset GS 3rd (2011) Imaging of cardiothoracic trauma in children – enigmas, edicts and errors. Pediatr Radiol 41(1 suppl):S67–S68
4. Balci AE, Kazez A, Eren S, Ayan E, Ozalp K, Eren MN (2004) Blunt thoracic trauma in children: review of 137 cases. Eur J Cardiothorac Surg 26(2):387–392

5. Renton J, Kincaid S, Ehrlich PF (2003) Should helical CT scanning of the thoracic cavity replace the conventional chest x-ray as a primary assessment tool in pediatric trauma? An efficacy and cost analysis. J Pediatr Surg 38:793–797
6. Anderson SW, Lucey BC, Varghese JC et al (2006) Sixty-four multi-detector row computed tomography in multitrauma patient imaging: early experience. Curr Probl Diagn Radiol 35(5):188–198
7. Patel RP, Hernanz-Schulman M, Hilmes MA, Yu C, Ray J, Kan JH (2010) Pediatric chest CT after trauma: impact on surgical and clinical management. Pediatr Radiol 40(7):1246–1253
8. Restrepo R, Lee EY (2012) Updates on imaging of chest wall lesions in pediatric patients. Semin Roentgenol 47(1):79–89
9. Körner M, Krötz MM, Degenhart C, Pfeifer KJ, Reiser MF, Lisenmaier U (2008) Current role of emergency US in patients with major trauma. Radiographics 28(1):225–242
10. Ding W, Shen Y, Yang J, He X, Zhang M (2011) Diagnosis of pneumothorax by radiography and ultrasonography: a meta-analysis. Chest 140(4):859–866
11. Coley BD (2011) Chest sonography in children: current indications, techniques, and imaging findings. Radiol Clin North Am 49:825–846
12. Pabon-Ramos WM, Williams DM, Strouse PJ (2010) Radiologic evaluation of blunt thoracic aortic injury in pediatric patients. Am J Roentgenol 194:1197–1203
13. Baker N, Woolridge D (2013) Emerging concepts in pediatric emergency radiology. Pediatr Clin North Am 60:1139–1151
14. Pearce MS, Salotti JA, Little MP et al (2012) Radiation exposure from CT scans in childhood and subsequent risk of leukaemia and brain tumours: a retrospective cohort study. Lancet 380(9840):499–505
15. Moore MA, Wallace EC, Westra SJ (2011) Chest trauma in children: current imaging guidelines and techniques. Radiol Clin North Am 49:949–968
16. Soldati G, Testa A, Silva FR et al (2006) Chest ultrasonography in lung contusion. Chest 130:533–538
17. Johnson NN, Toledo A, Endom EE (2010) Pneumothorax, pneumomediastinum and pulmonary embolism. Radiol Clin North Am 57:1357–1383
18. Westra SJ, Wallace EC (2005) Imaging evaluation of pediatric chest trauma. Radiol Clin North Am 43:267–281
19. Lomoschitz FM, Eisenhuber E et al (2003) Imaging of chest trauma: radiological patterns of injury and diagnostic algorithms. Eur J Radiol 48:61–70
20. Manson D, Babyn PS, Palder S et al (1993) CT of blunt chest trauma in children. Pediatr Radiol 24(1):1–5
21. Kirkpatrick AW, Sirois M, Laupland KB et al (2004) Hand-held thoracic sonography for detecting post-traumatic pneumothoraces: the extended focused assessment with sonography for trauma (EFAST). J Trauma 57:288–295
22. Soldati G, Testa A, Sher S, Pignataro G, La Sala M, Gentiloni Silveri N (2008) Occult traumatic pneumothorax: diagnostic accuracy of lung ultrasonography in the emergency department. Chest 133:204–211
23. Ianniello S, Di Giacomo V, Sessa B, Miele V (2014) First-line sonographic diagnosis of pneumothorax in major trauma: accuracy of E-Fast and comparison with multidetector computed tomography. Radiol Med. [Epub ahead of print]
24. Moore MA, Wallace EC, Westra SJ (2009) The imaging of paediatric thoracic trauma. Pediatr Radiol 39:485–496
25. Lee EY, Restrepo R, Dillman JR et al (2012) Imaging evaluation of pediatric trachea and bronchi: systematic review and updates. Semin Roentgenol 47(2):182–196
26. Dyer DS, Moore EE, Mestek MF et al (1999) Can chest CT be used to exclude aortic injury? Radiology 213:195–202

Abdominal Trauma

4

Margherita Trinci, Barbara Sessa, Guendalina Menichini, Viola Valentini, and Vittorio Miele

4.1 Introduction

Blunt trauma is the main cause of mortality and morbidity in pediatric patients; the abdomen is the second most common site of injury. As in an adult, there are two separate conditions according to the dynamics of the trauma that request different management: high- and low-energy trauma.

In high-energy trauma, a multiorgan involvement must be considered, studying not only the abdomen but also the head, chest, and limbs. The most frequent causes of high-energy trauma, just like in adults, are vehicle accidents, car vs. pedestrian accidents, and falls; but these causes vary according to age: toddlers are concerned with home traumas, children undergo sports trauma, and teenagers are involved in vehicle road accidents.

In low-energy trauma, a single organ/site must be considered. The most frequent causes of pediatric injury are those caused during sports activity, at school and at home.

A completely different evaluation is necessary in the case of a "beaten" child, which is discussed in another chapter.

The clinical anamnestic exam and the triage of the child may appear very difficult, in relation to the patient's age or in case of unconsciousness. At the first evaluation of the patient, the presence of bruises or wounds, together with blood and urine exams, can help to indicate the degree of the trauma.

Thus, diagnostic imaging plays an important role in the complex evaluation of the injured child.

In low-energy trauma and in isolated trauma, the first diagnostic approach in the child can be performed by X-ray, if needed, and ultrasound (US).

M. Trinci (✉) • B. Sessa • G. Menichini • V. Valentini • V. Miele
Cardiovascular and Emergency Radiology Department, S. Camillo Hospital,
C.ne Gianicolense, 87, Rome 00152, Italy
e-mail: margherita.trinci@libero.it; barbara.sessa@tiscali.it;
guendalina.menichini@gmail.com; violavalentini@libero.it; vmiele@sirm.org

V. Miele, M. Trinci (eds.), *Imaging Trauma and Polytrauma in Pediatric Patients*,
DOI 10.1007/978-3-319-08524-1_4

Table 4.1 Diagnostic imaging flow chart in pediatric abdominal trauma

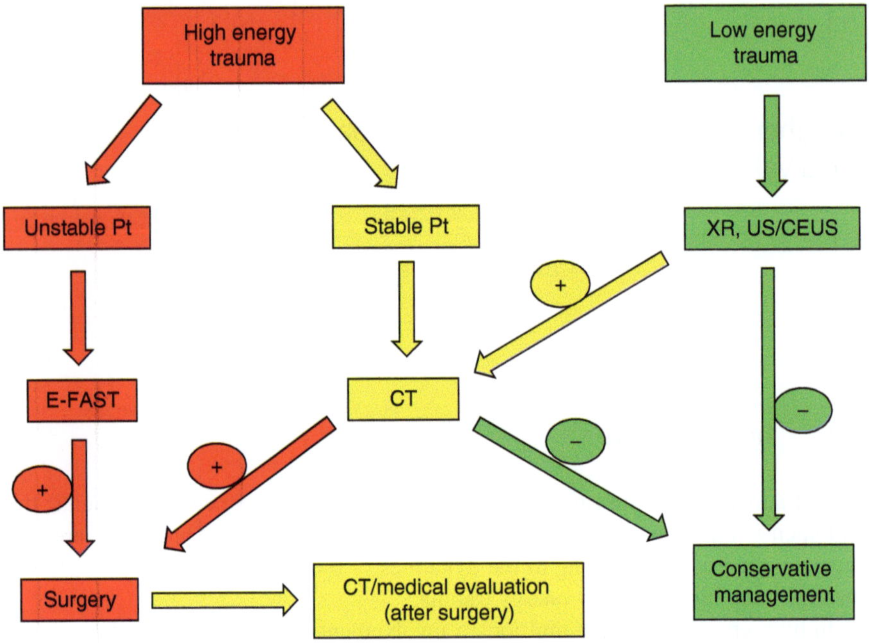

Ultrasound diagnostic accuracy is highly improved, thanks to the use of contrast-enhanced ultrasonography (CEUS) that increases the sensitivity and specificity of the given method.

In high-energy trauma, it is possible to have two different situations according to the severity of the clinical presentation, in particular of the hemodynamic condition (Table 4.1) [1–3].

In the hemodynamic unstable young patient, the first evaluation is performed through e-FAST, a rapid diagnostic method carried out during the first aid approach, which is necessary to depict the presence of hemothorax and pneumothorax and hemoperitoneum.

Should the hemodynamic stabilization occur, and in all stable patients with high-energy trauma, contrast-enhanced CT is performed, which is the gold standard in the evaluation of the injured patient.

After the initial evaluation and during follow-up procedures, the monitoring of an injured child must be performed according to radioprotection criteria, keeping in mind the patient's medical condition and laboratory exams [4, 5].

4.2 Ultrasound Technique

In high-energy blunt abdominal trauma, emergency US is performed in the emergency room on the unstable patient through e-FAST technique: the purpose is to depict the eventual hemoperitoneum in the four standard abdominal areas, right hypochondrium, left hypochondrium, epigastrium, and pelvis.

In fact, this technique has a high sensitivity, up to 99 % in literature review, in detecting abdominal free fluid even in small amounts. The aim of the exam is to depict in real time a huge hemoperitoneum that may be the cause of hemodynamic instability, which requests an immediate surgery. Therefore, the purpose of FAST is not the evaluation of abdominal parenchymal organs, which instead is carried out by means of computed tomography once hemodynamic stabilization is reached.

In low-energy or localized trauma, basic US is fundamental not only to evaluate the presence of hemoperitoneum but also to highlight parenchymal injuries.

For the latter purpose, US diagnostic efficiency has highly increased with the use of second-generation blood pool contrast agent, performing the contrast-enhanced ultrasound (CEUS). CEUS is much more sensitive than basic ultrasound in depicting parenchymal injuries and in the evaluation of their extension. In fact, CEUS has sensitivity and specificity values very similar to those of CT, which is the gold standard. Furthermore, it can depict active bleeding as a negative prognostic factor even if in a less accurate way as to CT.

The examination, for which it is necessary to obtain the parents' informed content, consists in the injection of US contrast medium, made up of a 2.4 ml suspension of phospholipid microbubbles of an inert gas (sulfur hexafluoride), through an antecubital vein followed by a bolus of 10 ml of physiological solution. Some specific elements are very important to carry out this procedure: to obtain the correct formation of microbubbles, the suspension should be shaken for at least 40 s and the injection should be done with at least an 18G needle; the use of smaller cannula needles, e.g., 20G, can destroy up to 20 % of the bubbles. After the injection, a rapid sequence exploration is done starting from the kidneys, then the liver, and ending with the spleen. The overall time needed is around 5 min (Fig. 4.1).

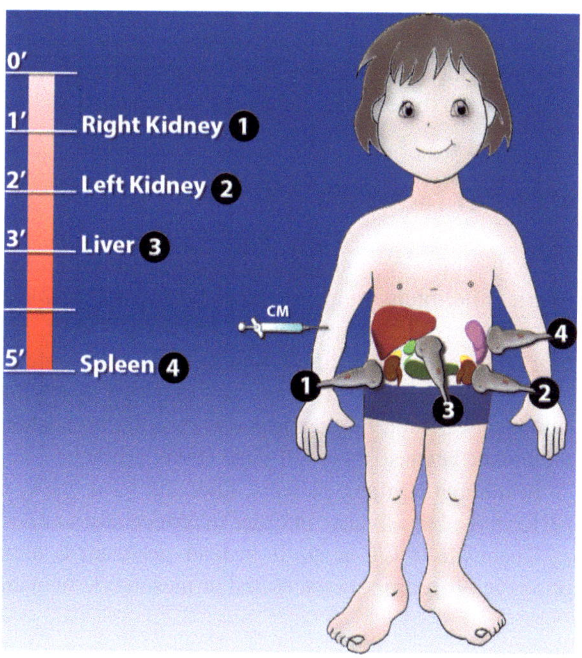

Fig. 4.1 CEUS protocol. CEUS exploration sequence: the kidneys, the liver, and finally the spleen

The US contrast medium elimination is rapid: after around 15 min, all the microbubbles break and the sulfur is eliminated through the lungs. US contrast medium has no nephrotoxic effect, and it is not metabolized by the kidney because it does not pass in the interstitial space, but it remains in the vessels.

Adverse reactions occur very rarely; severe reactions to the US contrast medium are not reported in pediatric patients in the literature.

At CEUS exam, the aspect of normal parenchyma is homogeneously hyperechoic; traumatic lesions appear as hypo-anechoic areas of different sizes and more or less defined, with or without capsular interruption, with morphology and extension corresponding to the CT exam.

The partial or total lack of enhancement of an organ is related to a vascular injury. The flow of contrast medium microbubbles out of the injured organ is due to extraparenchymal active bleeding. The presence of microbubbles in the damaged area can suggest intralesional blush.

It is possible and correct to administer a second dose of US contrast medium to solve any type of diagnostic doubt.

US and CEUS main benefits concern different aspects, as to its rapid performance, accuracy, and the possibility of avoiding unnecessary CT exams, thus reducing radio-exposure risks.

Besides the radioprotection aspects, US is ideal for pediatric use since a child has a higher quantity of water and a lower quantity of fat in his body as to an adult, so US imaging is of a higher quality in children than in adults.

CEUS limits are the same as those of basic US: the built of the patient, the presence of pneumoperitoneum, the presence of cutaneous wounds, and the evaluation of hemoretroperitoneum, together with the background experience knowledge and skills of the radiologist.

Furthermore, CEUS has specific limits in the evaluation of abdominal organs, in particular in depicting hollow viscera lesions, intestinal and mesenteric traumatic lesions, urinary tract injury, and the presence of active bleeding, as it has lower sensibility to the contrast-enhanced CT exam [6–9].

4.2.1 CT Technique

CT is the imaging method of choice in the evaluation of abdominal and pelvic injuries after blunt trauma in hemodynamically stable children.

In patients with major trauma, when the type of injury is not yet identified, it is best not to apply a specific-organ technique but a method which can show in detail any type of injury. CT scans are obtained from the lower chest to the pubic symphysis. Monitoring devices and metallic leads should be moved from the scanning plane because they will yield streak artifacts.

In traumatic young patients, after the scout view, it would be preferred not to perform the basal phase, in order to reduce radio-exposure.

Unenhanced CT scan, if instead performed, allows to highlight abdominal presence of free air, parenchymal or mesenteric hematoma, and bone fractures.

Imaging study with oral contrast medium administration is not recommended, due to the little advantage compared to the complexity of its administration in major trauma patients.

A 3-mm-thickness scan allows to perform good-quality imaging and subsequent good-quality reconstructions without excessive radiation exposure.

The intravenous iodine contrast medium volume depends on the patient's weight (approximately 2 ml/kg).

The CT technique has two contrast-enhanced phases: an arterial phase which is extended to all the body, to depict vascular injury or active bleeding, and an abdominal portal phase, to evaluate parenchymal and hollow viscera injury.

In the suspect of urinary tract injury, if the patient's clinical conditions are favorable, a later phase after 5 min is performed.

On the contrary, in case of suspected bladder injury, a retrograde distension with air may allow better visualization of the wall injury, especially in the anterior wall.

CT exam must always be completed with bidimensional reconstructions, on sagittal and coronal images, which are a fundamental help in understanding the extent of the injury. For bone component evaluation, 3D reconstructions with volume rendering (VR) can be used [10, 11].

4.3 Physiopathology

The continuous growth of the developing pediatric patient's body and the anatomical and structural differences with that of an adult are the main causes of the diversity of lesions and differences in the management between adult and child.

Whatever high-energy trauma occurs to a child, it is to be considered a potential cause of multiorgan lesions: this is why an equal impact force will determine a major impact area on a child due to the smaller body dimension compared to an adult.

A child reports less frequently bone fractures (e.g., ribs), due to a major flexibility in the bone structure of his body. This is why the absence of bone fractures does not imply a low-level energy impact, whereas the presence of bone fractures confirms a high-level energy trauma.

Besides, the protection provided by the lower ribs on abdominal parenchymal organs in the child is lower, both for the major flexibility of the ribs and for the relatively bigger dimension of the liver, spleen, and kidneys which protrude from the ribs, thus being directly exposed to the impact. The diaphragm muscle itself, which is in a more horizontal position, pushes down the liver and the spleen contributing in the protrusion from the ribs.

Other differences are the fact that the abdominal wall is thinner, due to the reduced muscle development, thus less adept in protecting in case of impact; there is less fat tissue in both subcutaneous abdominal tissue and in the intra-abdominal site, where it wraps parenchymal organs and all structures, partially absorbing the impact of the energy involved.

Ureters are wider and less tonic due to poor development of muscular tunic; the bladder is in a higher position because the pelvis is smaller and almost completely occupied by the rectus. Furthermore, the bladder which is intraperitoneal in the first years of life tends to descend in the pelvic area and to become retroperitoneal.

In the management of traumatic pediatric patient, nonoperative strategy is highly performed with respect to an adult patient, thus requesting surgery only if strictly needed.

Nonoperative management is ideal for pediatric patients as blood vessels are smaller with respect to an adult, and there is a major vasoconstrictive response, so visceral organ bleeding tends to be self-limited despite the severity of trauma.

At present, the choice of considering surgery is not strictly linked to the severity of the lesions or to the number of organs involved but to the capacity to normalize the hemodynamic condition despite all the pharmacological therapy in a maximum range of 6 h.

The liver, bowel, and spleen are highly vascularized organs within the peritoneal cavity, so there is a risk of a heavy bleeding. In all issues, active bleeding is a sign of severity and alarm, but still it does not mean that surgery is needed if hemodynamic values are normal.

Only bowel lesions always need surgery due to the high risk of bacterial contamination in the peritoneal cavity in case of traumatic perforation, not like parenchymal lesions.

As to the clinical outcome, we can say that in pediatric patients, hepatic lesions have a slower recovery as to spleen lesions, and multiorgan lesions have a slower recovery compared to isolated lesions.

4.4 Liver

Hepatic lesions are to be found in 10–30 % of blunt abdominal trauma; in many statistics, the liver is considered to be the organ which is mostly involved [12], both with isolated lesions and with lesions involving other organs, mainly the spleen. Lesions are often asymptomatic, and in 70 % of the cases, they can be treated in a nonoperative way. For anatomical reasons linked to coronary ligaments that hold the liver, the most exposed areas are the left lobe posterior segments which hit against the ribs and the dorsolumbar vertebral bodies.

Hepatic parenchymal lesions can extend and involve biliary ducts and blood vessels. Hemoperitoneum is present in around 2/3 of the cases and occurs if the lesion involves the organ capsule; if the capsule is saved, the hematoma will be intraparenchymal and/or subcapsular.

When the lesion involves the posterior surface of the liver which is not wrapped by the peritoneum, the so-called nude area, the blood expansion will occur in the retroperitoneal space. The consequent hemoretroperitoneum is usually located around the right adrenal gland and/or in the pararenal anterior space.

As in all organs, the most used classification of the severity range of hepatic lesions is that of the American Association for the Surgery of Trauma (AAST). This classification valid for both children and adults divides lesions in six categories, and it considers the type and extension of the parenchymal injury and the vascular involvement. Especially in pediatric patients, in whom the trauma management

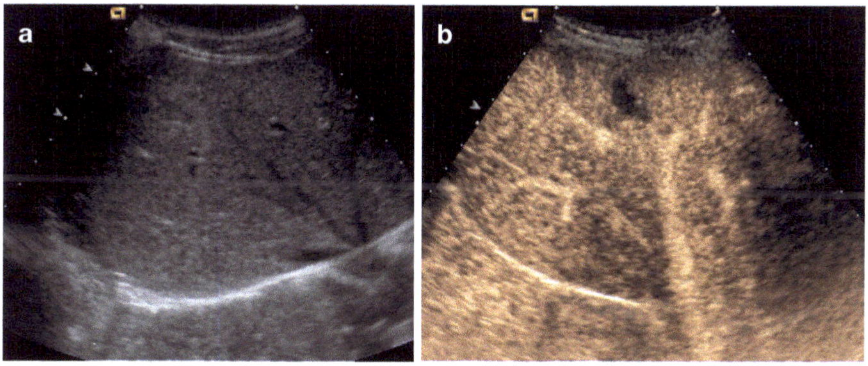

Fig. 4.2 A 10-year-old girl fell off the bicycle. Small hepatic tear. (**a**) US shows ill-defined hyperechoic area within VII hepatic segment. (**b**) CEUS well demonstrates a small anechoic laceration in the VII hepatic segment

tends to be nonoperative, the grading of parenchymal lesion is not the main factor in deciding the type of treatment to be performed, surgical or conservative. Other elements such as the hemodynamic stability and the multiorgan involvement determine the choice of the management. The severity of the lesion will determine the hospitalization period and the restrictions to be adopted after hospital discharge.

A shorter classification according to the traumatic lesion extension divides hepatic lesions in: minor, in case of less than 25 % of parenchyma injured in the involved lobe or in case of the presence of subcapsular hematoma; moderate, in case of values between 25 and 50 % of the involved lobe; and major, in case of more than 50 % of the lobe involved or in case of bilobar involvement [13].

4.4.1 US–CEUS

The right hypochondrium location immediately below the diaphragm, rib cage, and the intestinal gas cause an even more difficult US evaluation of hepatic dome and of the lateral segments, especially in patients that do not collaborate in breathing and correct positioning.

Even if in small amounts, the hemoperitoneum detection appears very clear, while hepatic lesion US evaluation, especially in the smallest lesions, can be difficult (Fig. 4.2).

Lesions can present different shapes, unclear borders, and iso-hyperechoic echostructure for the presence of fresh blood (Fig. 4.3). Subcapsular hematoma, as in CT, compresses the lateral margin of the hepatic parenchyma, and if very corpusculated, it can be difficult to differentiate from the normal parenchyma.

With CEUS the lesion will appear as an avascular area, hypo-anechoic compared to the normal hyperechoic parenchyma. In some cases, it is possible to see the presence of hyperechoic spots due to active bleeding in the anechoic lesion (Fig. 4.4).

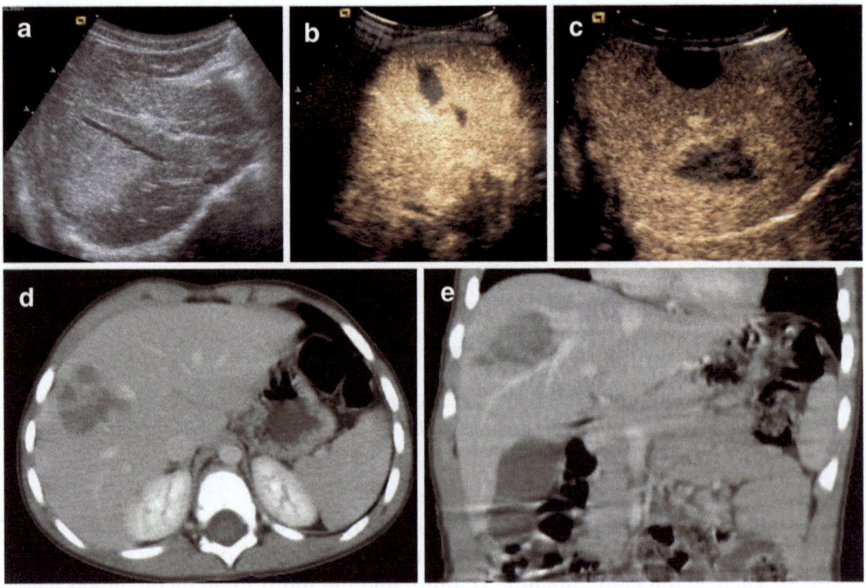

Fig. 4.3 A 4-year-old boy hit against a desk at school. Laceration with hematoma of the right hepatic lobe. (**a**) US, hyperechoic area in the right hepatic lobe. (**b**, **c**) CEUS, hypoechoic well-defined lesion. (**d**, **e**) Contrast-enhanced CT scan through upper abdomen shows irregular area with absence of contrast enhancement in the anterior segment of the right hepatic lobe. The images correspond to that of CEUS

In US follow-up, the size of the lesion will decrease, changing the echostructure from iso-hyperechoic to anechoic in time; even the hematomas will show the same echostructural changes together with the decrease in the size until the disappearance of the hematoma itself. With CEUS, the avascular area will show a progressive reduction in size and well-defined margins [6, 7, 9].

4.4.2 CT

The most frequent lesion is the parenchymal laceration. Contrast-enhanced CT shows a hypodense area, with a variable shape (Figs. 4.5 and 4.6). When the laceration reaches the capsular surface of the liver and breaks the Glissonian capsule, the hemoperitoneum always occurs; this is depictable through unenhanced CT scans, when performed immediately after trauma, as a high-density fluid, around 40 UH.

When the laceration does not reach the Glissonian capsule, hematoma occurs; it can be intraparenchymal and/or subcapsular. When intraparenchymal hematoma occurs, it is possible to depict it in basal phase CT, as a fuzzy hyperdense zone in the hepatic parenchyma, due to recent bleeding; after intravenous contrast medium administration, hematoma will appear hypodense compared to the normal enhanced parenchyma. Subcapsular hematoma typically compresses the lateral margin of the

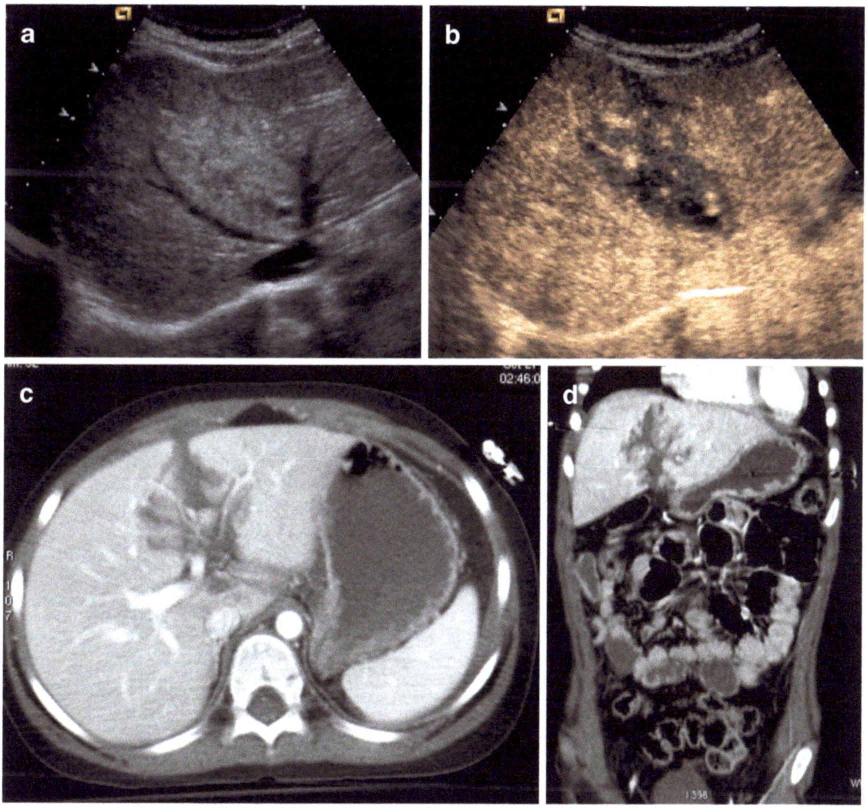

Fig. 4.4 A 14-year-old boy, sport trauma. Laceration of the IV hepatic segment with active bleeding. (**a**) US shows large hyperechoic area in the IV hepatic segment. (**b**) CEUS, hypoechoic lesion with hyperechoic spots suggestive of active bleeding. (**c**, **d**) Contrast-enhanced CT scan through upper abdomen shows irregular laceration with internal blush of contrast medium according to active bleeding

hepatic parenchyma, thus allowing an easier differential diagnosis compared to the perihepatic fluid (Fig. 4.7).

To carry out a prognostic evaluation, it is important to search for active bleeding in the hepatic lesion or in the hematoma, which appears as arterial phase contrast medium blush, eventually followed by a pooling in later phases (Fig. 4.8).

Traumatic hepatic vascular lesions are rare in pediatric patients. Avascular segments will appear hypodense after intravenous contrast medium administration. When post-traumatic hepatic artery pseudoaneurysm is seen through CT as hyperdense focus in the arterial phase within hepatic laceration, it is necessary to stress the issue and suggest the correct management through emergency embolization, even in the case of hemodynamic stability, as there is a high risk of rupture (around 80 %) [14].

The significance of periportal low hypodensity zones has been a matter of discussion; they have been considered a specific sign of hepatic trauma in the past. In fact, this issue is not only appreciable in traumatic lesions, and it seems to be linked

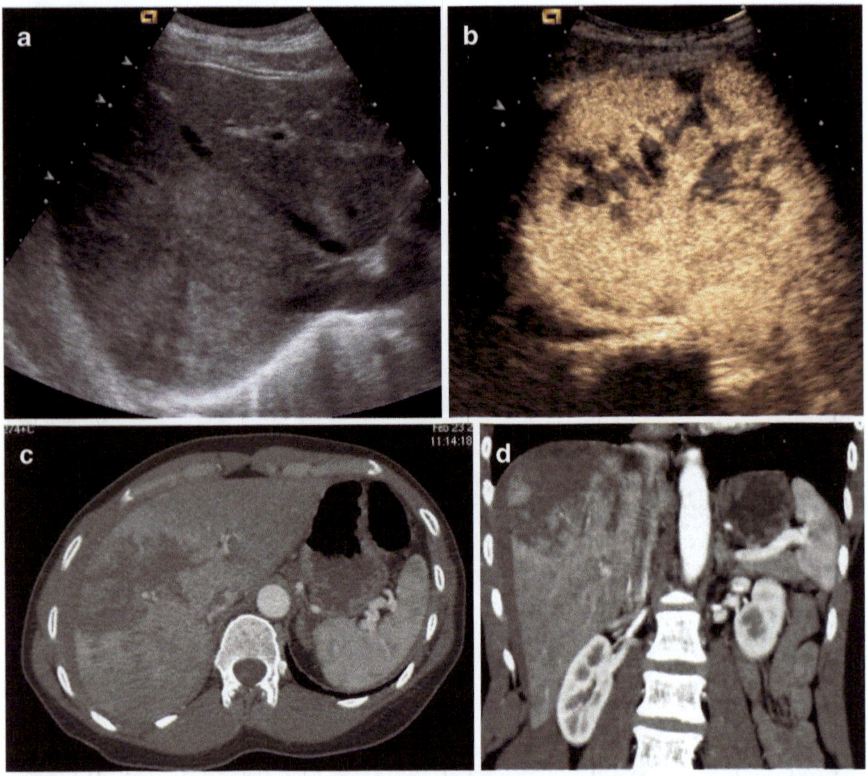

Fig. 4.5 A 17-year-old young girl. Trauma from falling off a horse during horse race. Ill-defined laceration of the liver. (**a**) US, irregular hyperechoic area in the right lobe. (**b**) CEUS shows multiple anechoic lacerations in the right hepatic lobe. (**c, d**) Contrast-enhanced CT confirms the presence of huge lacerations with irregular shape

not only to a specific organ lesion but to an overflow in lymphatic vessels in periportal spaces, due to a sudden increase in central venous pressure caused by too much fluid provided during the rescue phase.

During the follow-up, lesions treated nonoperatively after 1 month appear hypodense, due to reabsorbing of the corpusculated component; they gradually reduce their volume, usually to complete resolution, eventually leaving a small parenchymal cyst or a calcification.

It has been verified that usually minor and moderate lesions heal completely in 3–6 months while major lesions can remain even after 8–15 months. Subcapsular hematoma heals in around 2 months [13].

Complications in hepatic trauma are rare, they usually occur in the first month, and the clinical symptoms are fever, hypotension, peritonitis, etc. Other complications can be the abscessualization of the lesion in the first weeks, biloma that occurs between 12 days and 6 weeks (Fig. 4.9), hepatic artery pseudoaneurysm, subcapsular hepatic hematoma due to late bleeding, and choleperitoneum.

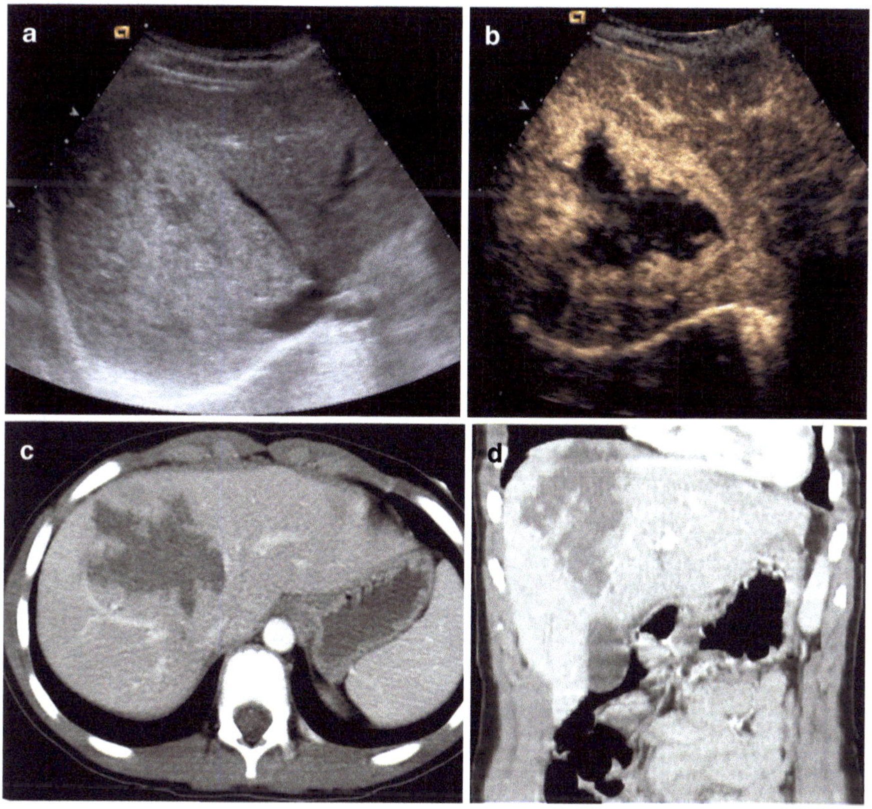

Fig. 4.6 A 9-year-old boy kicked by a horse. Laceration with hematoma of the right hepatic lobe. (**a**) US shows inhomogeneous hyperechoic area in the right hepatic lobe. (**b**) CEUS well defines the size and shape of the lesion, showing a large hypoechoic area. (**c**, **d**) Contrast-enhanced CT scan through upper abdomen shows irregular area with absence of contrast enhancement in the anterior segment of the right hepatic lobe, corresponding to that of CEUS

4.5 Spleen

The spleen is an intraperitoneal organ located in the abdominal left upper quadrant. It is the most vascularized organ of the body, in fact around 350 l of blood flow through it every day; this is why its injury is a potential risk for life, exposing the patient to a massive hemoperitoneum. While in adults the spleen is partially protected by the rib cage, in children, it is bigger, and for this reason, it protrudes and it is often involved in blunt abdominal trauma, with a frequency of 25 % of the cases both as isolated lesion and as multiorgan lesions.

The spleen is an important organ for the development and correct functioning of the immune system, especially in pediatric patients. Therefore, it is particularly important to perform the conservative treatment in traumatic splenic lesions [15–17].

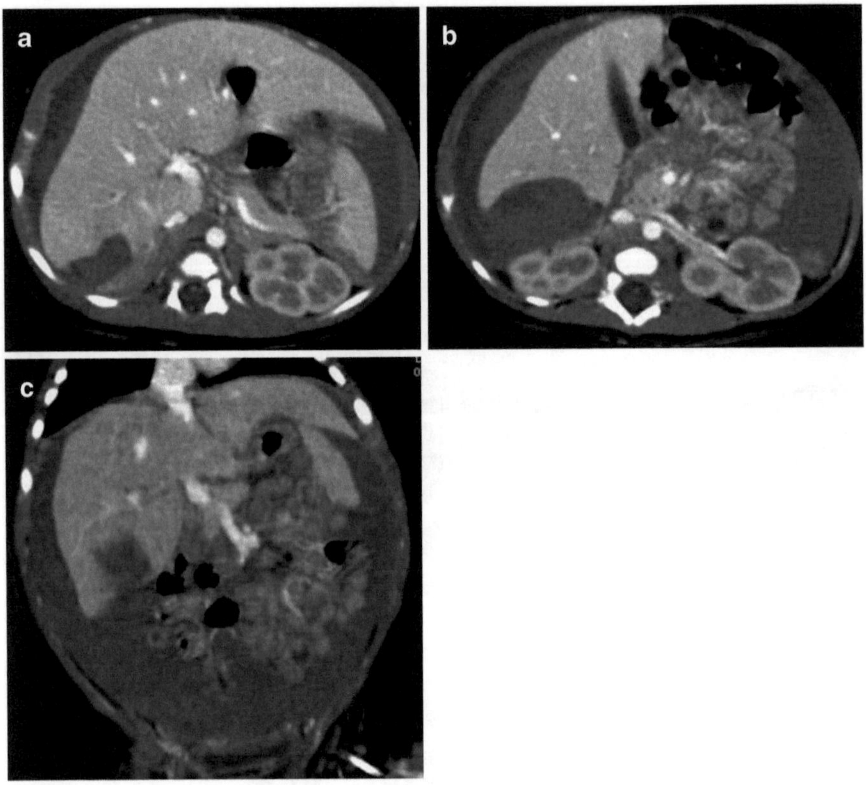

Fig. 4.7 Newborn with laceration and subcapsular hematoma of the liver. (**a**–**c**) Contrast-enhanced CT scan through upper abdomen shows laceration of the liver with associated subcapsular hematoma and large amount of hemoperitoneum

Imaging plays a fundamental role in differentiating the minor trauma, in which the observation of the patient is allowed, from those complex traumas which request immediate surgery.

Even for splenic lesions, as for hepatic lesions, the most used injury severity classification is that of AAST. As already said for the liver, this classification is not directly linked to the need of an operative management. In fact, if the patient is hemodynamically stable, despite hemoperitoneum or self-limited bleeding, the conservative management of the patient is recommended, considering its advantages, both because the immune function of the organ is preserved and because early and late complications caused by surgery are prevented, shortening hospitalization. Hemodynamic instability or the possibility of its happening is the main factor to perform splenectomy.

Splenic injuries have different shapes, linear or branched or complex; they can be associated to the presence of hemoperitoneum, in case of splenic capsula rupture, or to subcapsular or intraparenchymal hematoma, if the capsula is undamaged, around 25 % of cases [18].

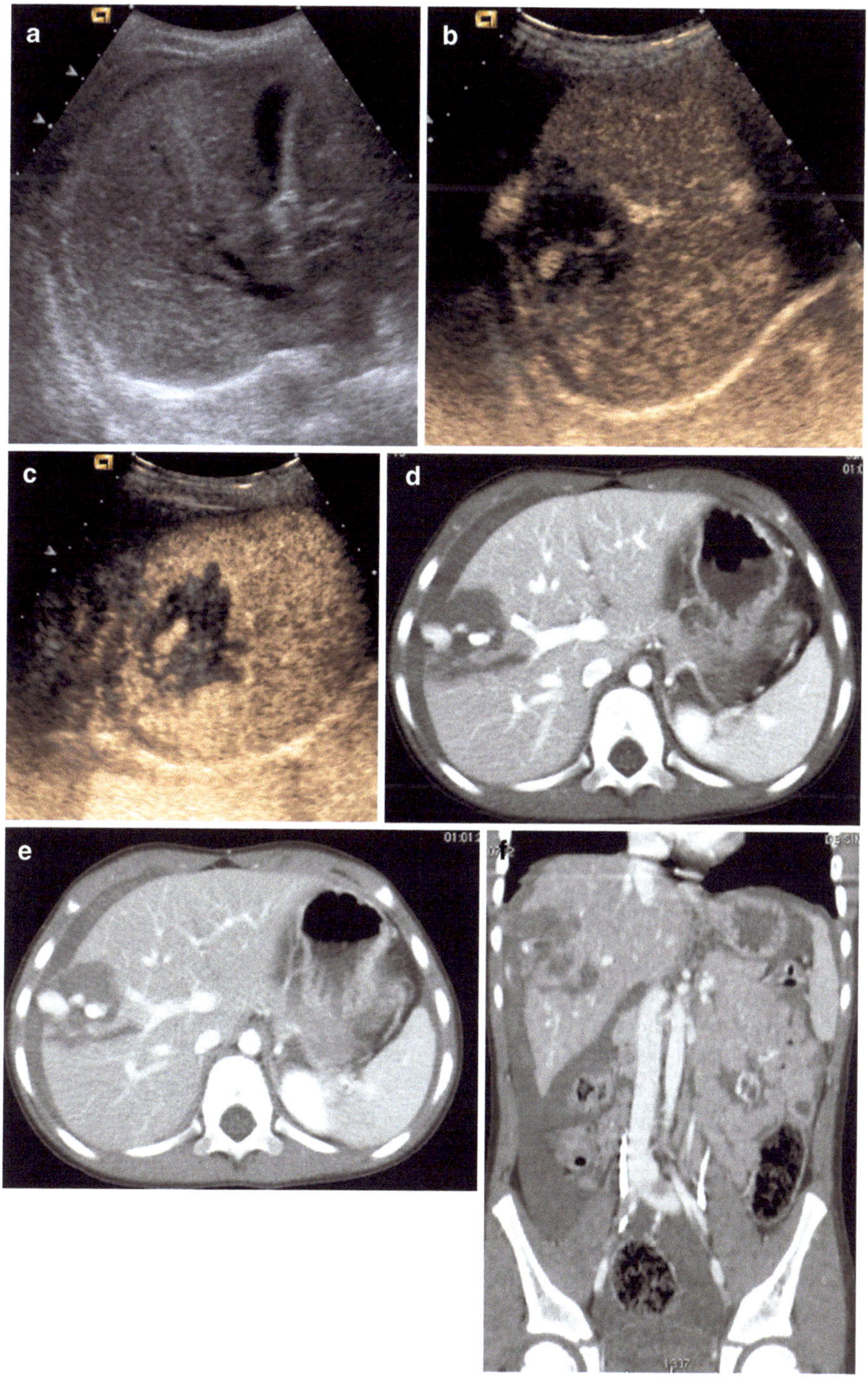

Fig. 4.8 A 6-year-old boy fell beating the right flank. Laceration of right the hepatic lobe with active bleeding. (**a**) US shows fuzzy hyperechoic area in the right hepatic lobe. (**b**, **c**) CEUS demonstrates hypoechoic lesion with hyperechoic large spots, both intralesional and extracapsular, due to active bleeding. (**d**, **e**) Contrast-enhanced CT scan through upper abdomen shows irregular tear with internal and extracapsular blush suggestive of active bleeding. Mild amount of hemoperitoneum is appreciable

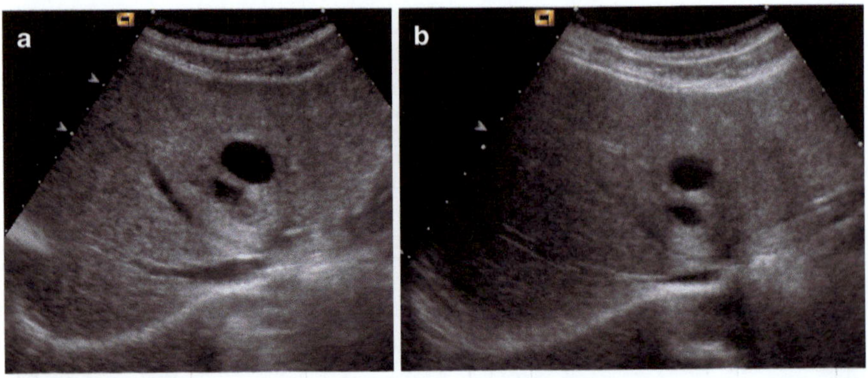

Fig. 4.9 Same patient of Fig. 4.4. Follow-up of hepatic laceration. Biloma. (**a**) US performed 1 month after trauma shows two fluid collections in the IV hepatic segments. (**b**) Follow-up US performed 3 months later shows the persistence of the rounded fluid collections, which appear to be related to bilomas

Hemoperitoneum linked to capsular lesion is most frequent when the hilum region is involved; furthermore, in this case, blood will flow along the splenorenal ligament at first, but then it will reach the retroperitoneum zone, in the anterior left pararenal space and around the pancreatic tail.

Two-time rupture of the spleen occurs rarely in adults, around 6 % of cases, and it is less frequent in children. It is a poor clinical evolution of an unknown subcapsular hematoma or of a vascular lesion as arterial-venous fistula or pseudoaneurysm. Even the late rupture can be treated with a conservative method, following the same criteria already mentioned for acute rupture. There are no links between late rupture and the insufficient rest of the patient. Bed rest is necessary only until abdominal pain is reported, and then a 3-month period of limited physical activity is suggested before going back to a normal lifestyle.

The recovery of the organ is strictly related to the severity of the lesions, and it can range from 3 to 20 weeks for a shattered spleen. The conservative management, even if partial, is very important in the preservation of the immunological function of the spleen; studies carried out on adults have shown that immunological function is preserved if at least 1/3 of the parenchyma is saved.

Literature states that minor lesions (I and II level) can be considered self-healing and patients can leave the hospital just after a 1-day bed rest and start their normal daily functions except sports activity, which can be started again after 6 weeks.

In major trauma, hospitalization and bed rest can be 2–3 days; after, hemodynamically stable patient without pain can be discharged and must follow the above protocol. The patient will undergo a 6–10-week follow-up according to the severity of the lesion [19].

4.5.1 US–CEUS

The spleen is considered to be a difficult organ to be evaluated by US, especially the upper pole zone, located in the subphrenic region. US exam of the given region can be influenced by pulmonary air, and it is also difficult to perform due to the rib cage.

Fresh blood echogenicity is very similar to that of normal parenchyma; for this reason, it is possible to mistake traumatic lesion, even the largest. Often, the most evident sign of splenic lesion is the presence of a hypo-anechoic fluid collection in the subcapsular or perisplenic space.

Parenchymal lesions can be difficult to recognize (Fig. 4.10a); but when depicted, they are relatively hypoechoic as to the normal parenchyma. When no perisplenic fluid is reported, it can be very difficult to recognize the involvement of the capsular surface of the organ.

CEUS overcomes all these limits.

CEUS parenchymal lesion evaluation must be performed during the venous phase, 120–240 s after contrast medium injection, after its diffusion in the sinusoidal circle, when normal parenchyma shows a high homogeneous echogenicity which is absent in the arterial phase.

CEUS aspect of splenic lesions is always that of anechoic areas that are clearly highlighted as to normal hyperechoic parenchyma (Fig. 4.10b). The extension of the lesion to the splenic capsula and the capsular interruption is highly recognizable (Fig. 4.11a, b). Furthermore, subcapsular or perisplenic fluid is more visible due to the parenchymal contrast enhancement.

CEUS sensitivity in depicting splenic parenchymal lesions is very similar to that performed by CT, allowing a detailed follow-up even during the bed rest phase, without radiation exposure [6, 9].

4.5.2 CT

The sensitivity and specificity of CT in the detection of splenic injury is close to 100 %.

Splenic lesions are correctly shown at contrast-enhanced CT in the portal phase, when parenchyma is homogeneously and widely enhanced. Instead the splenic parenchyma has a mottled appearance in arterial phase CT scan; this can cause misinterpretations in the evaluation of the organ if examined at a too early stage.

Splenic lesions are usually represented by lacerations that can involve the parenchyma either partially or as full-thickness tear causing the complete fracture of the organ (Figs. 4.10c, d and 4.11c, d). Contusive lesions and intraparenchymal hematomas are rare and have lower severity, and they can appear even when no subcapsular or perisplenic fluid is reported. Cases of shattered spleen, which consists in the breaking of the organ in three or more fragments that go along with huge hemoperitoneum, can be clinically related to hemodynamic instability. These lesions are those that request urgent surgery as they represent a high death risk as a consequence of hemorrhagic shock.

Any deficiency in detection is usually a result of misinterpretation that can be related either to the evaluation of the organ in a non-appropriate phase or to preexisting nontraumatic lesions.

Even the presence of congenital clefts can lead to misinterpretation and false-positive patients. We have to consider that congenital clefts have regular and homogeneous well-defined profiles as to the lacerations that appear more irregular and are often linked to subcapsular and/or perisplenic fluid [18].

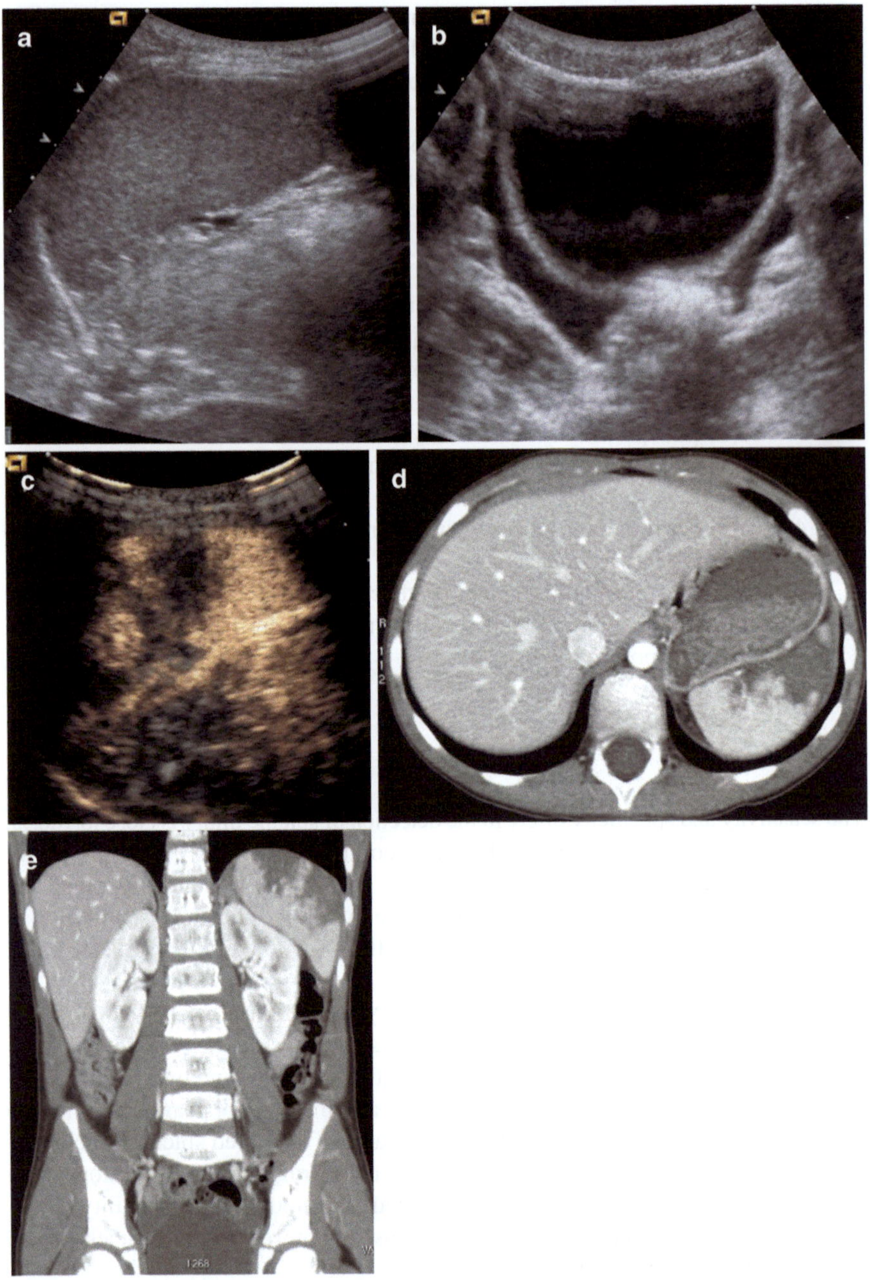

Fig. 4.10 A 9-year-old boy fell beating the left side on a wooden table. Splenic lesion. (**a**, **b**) US shows normal appearance of the spleen; free fluid in the pelvic space. (**c**) CEUS shows irregular anechoic areas in the spleen. (**d**, **e**) Contrast-enhanced axial and coronal CT show large hypodense parenchymal lesions, with absence of perisplenic fluid

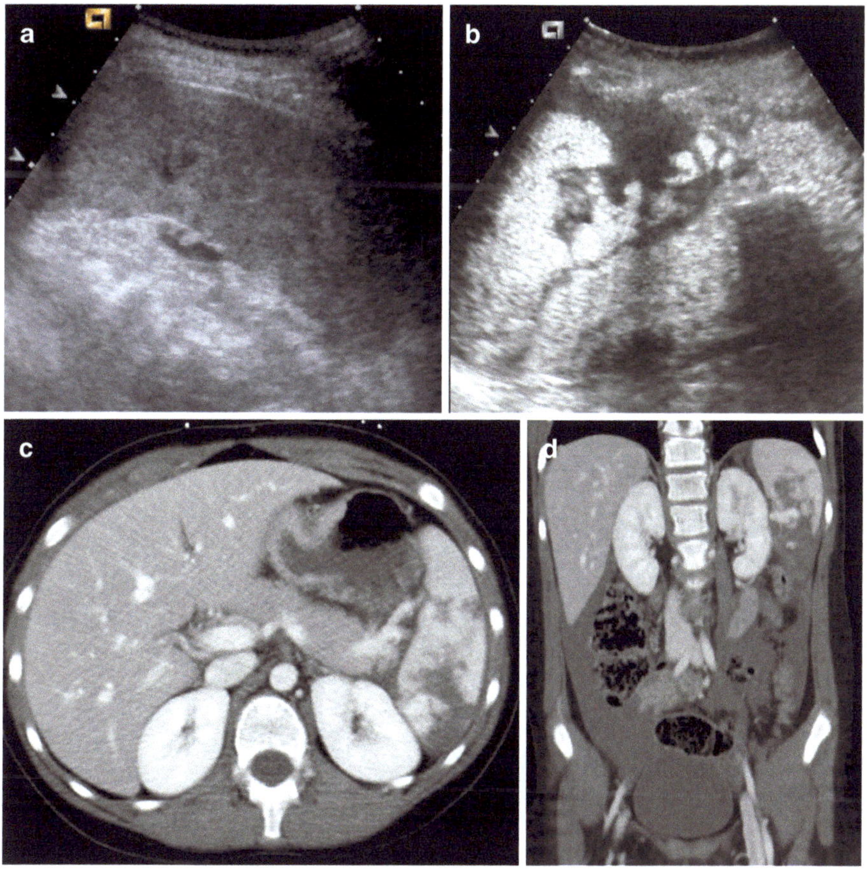

Fig. 4.11 A 10-year-old girl kicked by a horse. (**a**) US shows widespread inhomogeneity of the splenic parenchyma. (**b**) CEUS well demonstrates a large lesion of the lower pole with hyperechoic spots due to active bleeding. (**c**, **d**) Axial and coronal contrast-enhanced CT show shattered spleen with active bleeding in the lower pole and relevant hemoperitoneum

Besides being used in shattered spleen management, operative handling is performed in case of intraparenchymal active bleeding and especially in peritoneal cavity active bleeding (Fig. 4.12).

Instead, in case of vascular complications, such as arterial-venous fistula or post-traumatic pseudoaneurysm (Fig. 4.13), splenic artery embolization (SAE) can be performed with a selective or super selective technique according to angiographic results. Angiographic technique is reported to be more safe compared to surgery, and it has a mortality rate in the first 6 months of around 2.4 % compared to 8 %.

Among the most frequent morbidity causes after embolization, we can find pleural fluid effusion, pancreatitis due to embolization of collateral branches coming

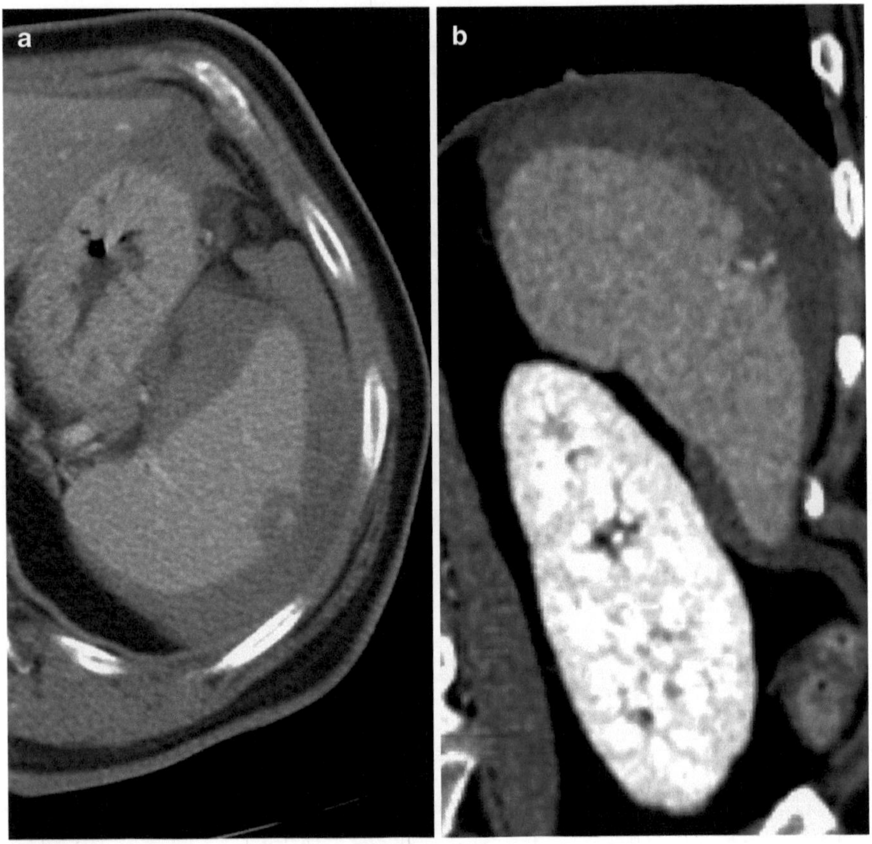

Fig. 4.12 A 16-year-old girl hit her left hip against a piece of furniture. Spleen lesion. (**a**, **b**) Contrast-enhanced CT shows little subcapsular lesion with extracapsular blush and hemoperitoneum

from spleen artery, and splenic abscesses. Morbidity and mortality are linked to a high percentage of embolized splenic tissue around 70 %; surgery is preferred when angiography implies a great loss of splenic tissue [15].

4.6 Urinary System: Kidneys, Urinary Tract, Bladder, and Urethra

Renal trauma is relatively frequent in children: the kidneys are the third most involved organ in blunt abdominal trauma. Urinary system lesions involve the kidney in 80 % of the cases, followed by the external genitals, bladder, urethra, and ureter.

In 75 % of the cases, kidneys are involved in multiorgan traumas, often blunt or contusive (85 %), less frequently open or penetrating (15 %).

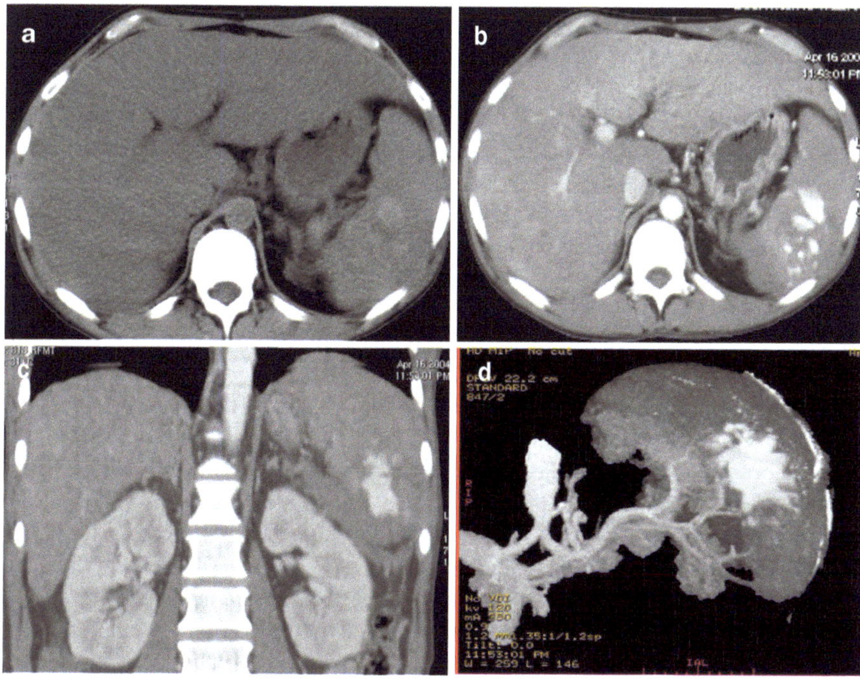

Fig. 4.13 A 16-year-old boy, street accident. AV fistula of the spleen. (**a**) Unenhanced CT scan shows hyperdense area in the central zone of the spleen. (**b, c**) Axial and coronal contrast-enhanced CT show intense opacification of large area of the splenic parenchyma. (**d**) VR 3D reconstruction demonstrates the relationship with hilar splenic vessels

Isolated trauma occurs most frequently in low-energy trauma (98 %) and can often be managed in a conservative way. In this case, the left kidney is involved more than the right kidney, because it protrudes from the lower ribs and it is less protected.

Operative management in isolated trauma is rarely needed, around 2 % of the cases.

Depending on the different type of impact force, lesions reported can involve the renal parenchyma, vascular system, or urinary system. Parenchymal lesions usually are the result of a direct impact, while decelerative forces cause vascular and/or urinary tract lesions.

Clinical evaluation of renal trauma in pediatric patients is often difficult, due to a nonspecific and unclear symptomatology. The typical and more specific symptom is hematuria. Gross hematuria is the most significant and characteristic clinical sign of renal trauma, found in more than 95 % of cases, but not always related to the severity of the trauma. In fact, hematuria can also be unrevealed in severe traumatic lesion as in 24 % of patients with renal artery thrombosis and in up to 1/3 of cases of pyeloureteral junction lesions. Gross hematuria is more frequent in penetrating trauma compared to blunt trauma, and it is rare in trauma due to deceleration force.

AAST classification divides renal trauma in five classes according to renal damage with parenchymal extension, to urinary system involvement, or to vascular pedicle injury.

More severe lesions (IV and V degree) are those that occur with urinary system damage and/or the arterial-venous vascular involvement, causing organ ischemia, with irreversible lesion.

Therefore, the classification is related to the development of the prognostic factors, allowing to differentiate patients with mild-to-moderate trauma (stages I–III), requesting normal clinical-radiological observation, from patients with severe trauma (stages IV–V), which require a surgical and/or interventional treatment.

The management of renal trauma in fact is often conservative; operative treatment is necessary in case of hemodynamically unstable patients or there is either a complete destruction of the pyeloureteral junction or a lesion on the artery or renal vein with devascularization of the kidney.

The correlation between a lesion and its severity also allows to get an idea of the recovery time of the patient. American literature limits the time of hospitalization, even in severe trauma, which depends primarily on hemodynamic conditions. The retroperitoneal position of the kidneys, which are enveloped by Gerota's fascia, causes a self-limited bleeding, as opposed to the organs placed in the peritoneal cavity. It is known that in localized trauma, painful symptoms stop in about a day and feeding is resumed by the second day after the trauma. The presence of hematuria does not influence the time of hospitalization. Microhematuria can be detected for more than a month also if the damage does not leave any sequelae. If the patient is able to void spontaneously, despite the injury, intravesical catheter is not needed [20].

4.6.1 US–CEUS

The injured kidney at US exam can appear normal or moderately swollen compared to the contralateral; sometimes there is a hyperechoic parenchymal zone suggesting traumatic lesion (Figs. 4.14a and 4.15a).

The presence of perirenal effusion appears as an anechoic area, which can vary in size, surrounding the kidney (Fig. 4.16a). US has a low sensitivity and low negative predictive value for the assessment of hemoretroperitoneum.

The use of CEUS significantly increases the sensitivity in detecting the parenchymal lesions, and perirenal hematoma, even if very small [9].

The kidneys are evaluated in the first 2 min after the infusion of the contrast agent. The evaluation is already performed in the arterial phase of parenchymal enhancement, but it is more accurate in the venous phase, in which the enhancement of the parenchyma appears more homogeneous.

At CEUS lesions appear as hypo-anechoic areas in the context of highly echogenic renal parenchyma (Figs. 4.14b and 4.15b). The perirenal fluid appears more evident due to the increased contrast compared to the enhanced parenchyma (Figs. 4.14b, 4.15b, c, and 4.16b). In case of traumatic vascular injury, the kidney appears partially or totally hypo-anechoic.

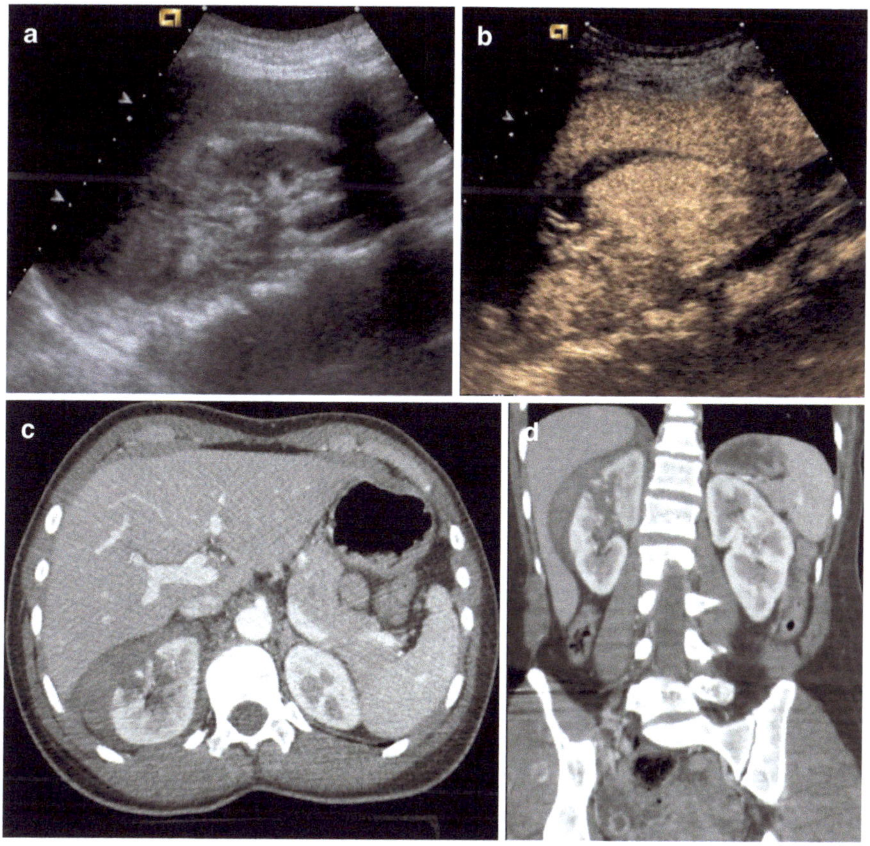

Fig. 4.14 A 16-year-old girl. Trauma caused by a crash between a car and a motorbike. Renal tear with active bleeding. (**a**) US shows inhomogeneous hyperechoic area of the upper pole of the right kidney. (**b**) CEUS shows a small tear of the kidney with small perirenal fluid and hyperechoic blush suggestive of active bleeding. (**c**, **d**) Axial and coronal contrast-enhanced CT confirm renal tear, active bleeding, and perirenal fluid

The limitations of CEUS are also represented by the incomplete assessment of the retroperitoneum, by the difficulty to detect active bleeding, and by the inability to highlight the injuries of the urinary tract, because, as already mentioned, the contrast agent is not excreted by the kidneys [6, 21].

4.6.2 CT

CT technique for kidneys is the same as that used in the study of other abdominal parenchymal organs, adding, however, when suspecting the lesion of the urinary tract, a delayed scan after contrast medium administration (about 5–10 min), in the excretory phase to demonstrate the leakage of iodinated urine.

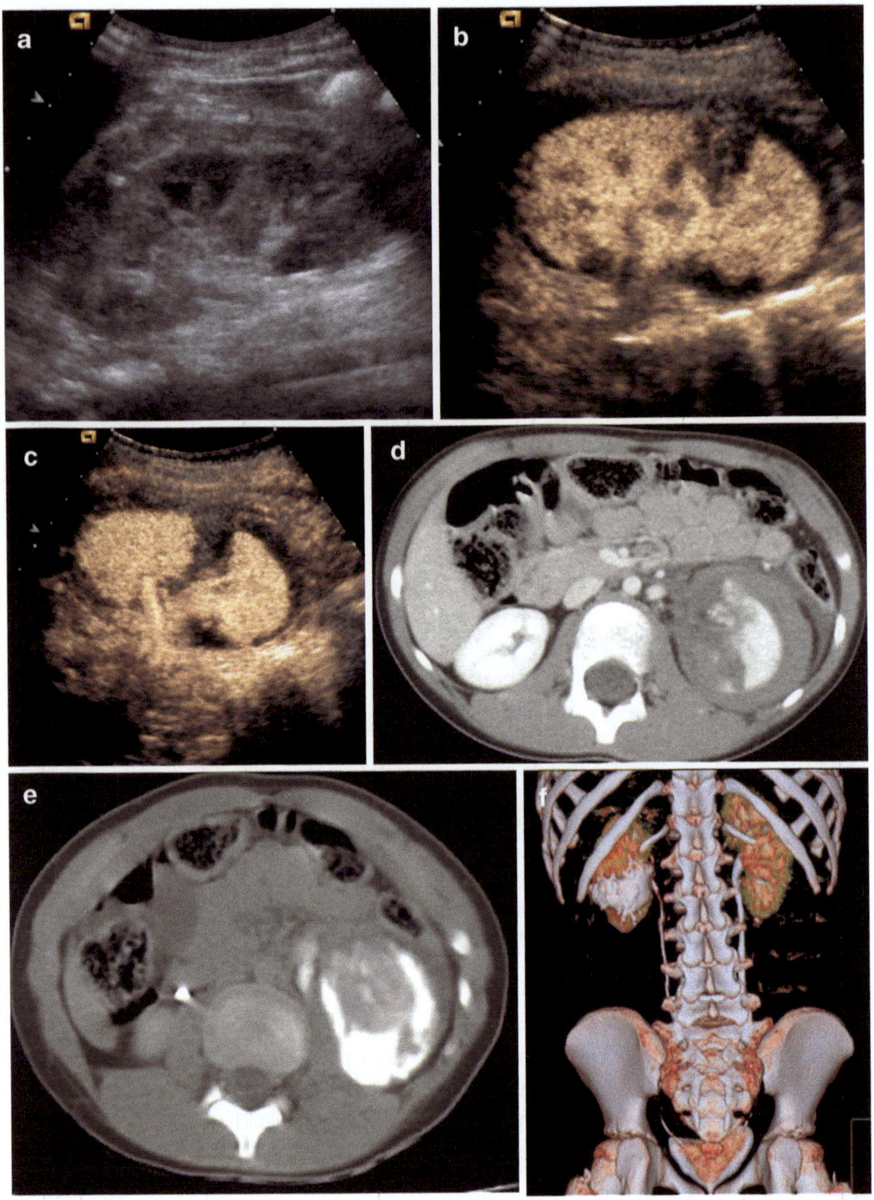

Fig. 4.15 A 10-year-old girl fell in the school playground and presents with hematuria. (**a**) US shows inhomogeneous hyperechoic area with hazy profiles of the upper pole of the right kidney, with small amount of perirenal fluid. (**b, c**) CEUS demonstrates deep laceration of the kidney, involving the parenchyma, suggesting the involvement of the urinary system; perirenal fluid. (**d–f**) Contrast-enhanced CT confirms the lesion shown by CEUS and in the late phase allows to demonstrate the perirenal contrast medium leakage due to urinoma

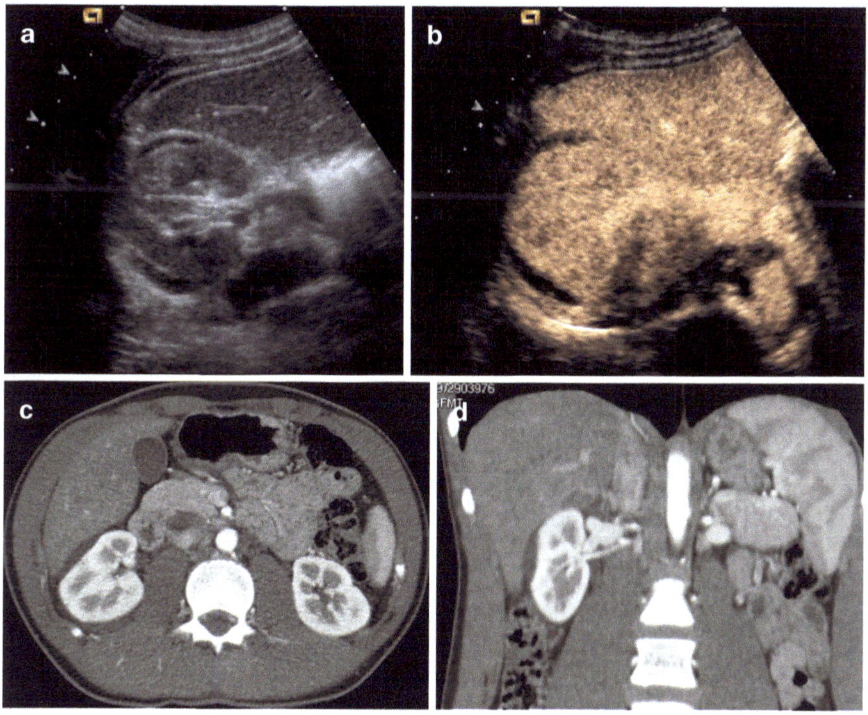

Fig. 4.16 A 14-year-old boy. Trauma occurring during a football game. Subcapsular renal hematoma. (**a**) US shows a subtle perirenal fluid collection. (**b**) CEUS well demonstrates the fluid collection that marks the cortical profile of the right kidney. (**c**, **d**) Contrast-enhanced CT confirms the findings of CEUS

The most common renal injury is the less severe and it is the parenchymal contusion; it represents a bruised organ characterized by microscopic areas of hemorrhage with edema. On CT the involved kidney may appear larger than the other kidney as a result of the associated edema. Before contrast medium injection, the renal contusion can be seen as a hyperintense parenchymal area; after contrast medium administration, it appears as a focal or diffuse region of delayed contrast enhancement.

Renal lacerations appear as linear low-attenuation areas in the parenchyma (Figs. 4.14c, d and 4.15d, e). The severity of the injury is linked to the extension of the lesion: the superficial lacerations are limited into the renal parenchyma, the deeper ones more likely involve the renal collecting system. Active bleeding can be detected within the tear.

Renal infarction is due to a main or segmental renal arterial branch laceration.

A segmental renal infarct occurs in case of injury to a segmental renal artery: at enhanced CT scan, it is like a peripheral wedged-shaped area of nonenhancing parenchyma. The management of renal segmental infarction is nonoperative and results in

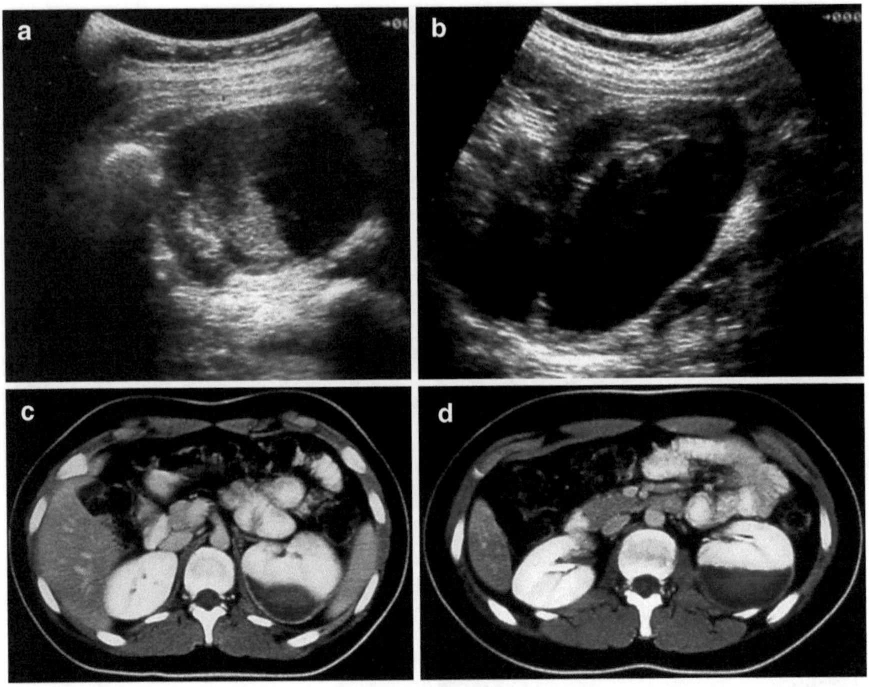

Fig. 4.17 A 16-year-old girl. Street accident. Subcapsular left kidney hematoma. (**a**, **b**) US shows a large amount of anechoic fluid that marks the renal parenchyma. (**c**, **d**) CT confirms the findings of US

a focal area of renal scarring. Injury to the main renal artery produces devascularization of the entire kidney. This is the most severe form of renal injury and must be treated promptly because permanent, progressive loss of renal function begins 2 h after trauma.

Subcapsular or perinephric hematoma can be found in any renal trauma. CT aspect is typical: a subcapsular hematoma is limited in its extension by the renal capsule, causing mass effect on renal profile (Fig. 4.17), whereas a perinephric hematoma is distributed throughout the perirenal space; if it is relevant, it can be dislocated to the kidney.

At the unenhanced CT scan, the hematoma is typically hyperintense, while it becomes hypointense after intravenous contrast medium administration (Fig. 4.15d). The assessment of any active bleeding in the early stages after contrast medium administration is very important (Fig. 4.14c, d); in fact in case of severe bleeding, the management of the patient changes from conservative to operative.

The assessment of any lesion of the urinary tract, as already mentioned, must be done with delayed scans. On CT images, renal collecting system injury results in urinary leakage of IV contrast medium (Fig. 4.15e, f).

Urine leakage typically remains contained in the perirenal space and is called as a “urinoma.” Seldom, urinary leakage and/or hemorrhage may reach the pelvis due to direct communication between the perirenal space in the abdomen and the prevesical extraperitoneal space in the pelvis. Usually the management of renal collecting system injury is nonoperative, mostly if the leak is confined to the perirenal space; sometimes, urinary tract obstruction requiring surgical repair may result.

4.7 Bladder and Urethra

Due to its anatomical position, well protected by the pelvic ring, injuries of the bladder are rare, occurring in 1–2 % of trauma patients, most commonly secondary to blunt trauma due to a high-energy injury. We have to remember that the bladder in children is considered an intraperitoneal organ in contrast to the adult where it is considered an organ mainly extraperitoneal.

Pelvic fractures, especially those in the pelvic ring, mostly the bilateral ones, are frequently associated, nearly 80–90 % of cases, with lower urinary tract injuries, though only 5–10 % of pelvic fractures result in bladder injury. The frequency of pelvic fractures in children presents a peak between 6 and 12 years of age and they are more frequent in males than in females.

The traumatic mechanisms are more frequently those in which high energy is transferred to the patient such as in pedestrian motor-vehicle accidents, falls from height, or crush injury and in trauma from the safety belt. The distention at the time of the trauma allows the rupture of the bladder.

In pelvic fracture, two mechanisms predominate as causes of bladder injury. The first involves shearing forces at deceleration resulting in injury at the fixed sites of pelvic fascial attachment. The second is caused by direct injury from pelvic bone fragments causing laceration of the bladder wall. Intraperitoneal blunt injury is due to rapid deceleration that determines a sudden increase of intravesical pressure, resulting in a "burst-type" injury.

Traumatic lesion starts from wall contusion to rupture. Bladder rupture can be both intraperitoneal or extraperitoneal, or combined.

In very young children, most of the injuries are intraperitoneal, because of the partial intra-abdominal location of the bladder.

Extraperitoneal bladder rupture occurs more frequently than intraperitoneal rupture in teenagers, and it is often caused by bone spicule of a pelvic fracture, pubic symphysis diastasis, sacral fractures, and sacroiliac joint diastasis.

Intraperitoneal rupture in teenagers is less frequent, around 20 %, and typically results from shearing of the distended bladder by a lap belt.

However, the overall incidence is lower because pelvic fracture is also lower in children; there is no relation between isolated acetabular fracture and the presence of bladder lesions. As opposed to adults, bladder neck injuries are more common in boys with a pelvic crush injury rather than urethral injuries as reported in adults.

Gross hematuria is believed to be associated with more significant injuries, as in the case of rupture, while microhematuria has been more commonly related to bladder contusion.

In addition to hematuria that is present in approximately 90 % of bladder trauma, the inability to void or suprapubic pain may occur.

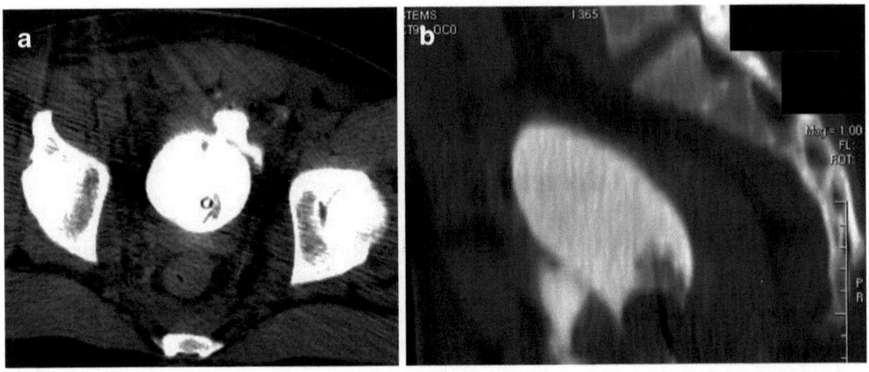

Fig. 4.18 A 16-year-old boy. Motorbike vs. car. Extraperitoneal bladder rupture. (**a**, **b**) Axial and sagittal contrast-enhanced CT in the delayed phase show the rupture of the anterior wall of the bladder, with the leakage of iodinated urine in the extraperitoneal pelvic space

Imaging of the bladder, if indicated, may consist of cystography and is performed in the clinically stable patient. CT cystography is performed more liberally because of the central role of CT scanning in trauma assessment.

CT has 95 % sensitivity and 100 % specificity in the detection of bladder rupture; some studies point to a lower accuracy in intraperitoneal rupture, with sensitivity and specificity values of 80 and 99 %.

For CT cystography, the bladder is filled retrograde with contrast medium, and the scan is performed after 300–400 mL of contrast is instilled.

Extraperitoneal contrast leakage is confined to the pelvis on CT and appears as a "flame-shaped" opacity (Fig. 4.18). Characteristic patterns of intraperitoneal contrast leakage include pooling in the cul-de-sac, paracolic gutter, or retrohepatic space on CT or outlining of bowel loops.

Another way to evaluate the integrity of the bladder through CT exam is through retrograde gas distension. The advantage is the easier air distribution which allows, even in the absence of an overdistension of the bladder, to hypothesize the presence of a rupture, through the flow of extraluminal air bubbles, even in the case of small lesions or lesions located on the anterior wall.

Most extraperitoneal bladder injuries can be managed conservatively with catheter drainage; in other cases, such as for penetrating injuries, surgery is requested.

Traumatic lesions of the urethra are, for anatomical reasons, more frequent in males.

Female urethral injuries are uncommon, 0–6 %, because the urethra itself is very short, and usually, all involved injuries are associated with pelvic fracture as a result of laceration by bone fragments.

Anatomically, the urethra is divided into anterior and posterior segments.

The clinical suspicion in male is given by gross blood at the urethral meatus and/or scrotal hematoma while in female is given by vaginal bleeding, pelvic fracture and bleeding, perineal ecchymosis, and pelvic fracture.

The mechanism of injury varies depending on the anterior urethral segment injuries and is the result of blows to the perineum. Posterior urethral injuries are often associated with pelvic fracture. When gross blood is present at the urethral meatus, retrograde urethrography (RUG) is indicated before catheterization; if blind catheter placement is performed, a partial injury can accidentally become a complete injury.

Early management of most posterior urethral injuries involves urinary diversion with a suprapubic catheter. Urethral lesions are classified in five grade groups. Grades I and II urethral injuries can be managed without catheterization, if the patient is able to void. Partial anterior injuries are managed with a urethral catheter alone, and a pericatheter urethrogram is performed at 7–10 days to confirm healing before its removal. Most posterior injuries can be managed with urinary diversion and delayed (3–6 months) reconstruction, following resorption of the pelvic hematoma.

Endoscopic techniques of primary realignment show promise in potentially decreasing the rates of stricture formation while providing equivalent results with regard to continence and erectile dysfunction.

4.8 Pancreas

Pancreatic trauma is less common because of the deep position of the organ, relatively protected by the abdominal wall and the surrounding fat. In a child, however, this protection is less effective than in an adult, due to the reduced development of the muscle wall and the relatively poor quantity of superficial and deep adipose tissue.

Pancreatic trauma happens in 3–12 % of blunt abdominal trauma; it rarely occurs as isolated injury, but usually 60 % of cases are associated with lesions of the liver, spleen, or duodenum. This means that in patients with pancreatic lesions, morbidity and mortality increase.

Diagnosis is essential, even for prognostic purposes. The detection of lesions limited to the parenchyma may allow conservative treatment, while in case of duct injury the management depends on the site of the lesion. If the distal portion on the left side of the spine (grade III) is involved, duct stenting or surgery for partial resection of the pancreas is needed; surgical treatment is definitive with acceptable operative risk; surgical therapy allows for a shorter recovery compared to the unoperated patient with ductal injury. The lesions in the proximal part of the duct are of greater severity (grade IV), but surgical treatment is more complex for the deep location of these lesions; for this reason they are managed more often by the positioning of a stent, preventing surgery.

Pancreatic trauma is the leading cause of pancreatitis in children [22, 23].

4.8.1 US

Because of its deep position and the interposition of intestinal gas content, the pancreas is a difficult organ to evaluate through US exam; however, in children the evaluation is easier, mainly because of their physical structure.

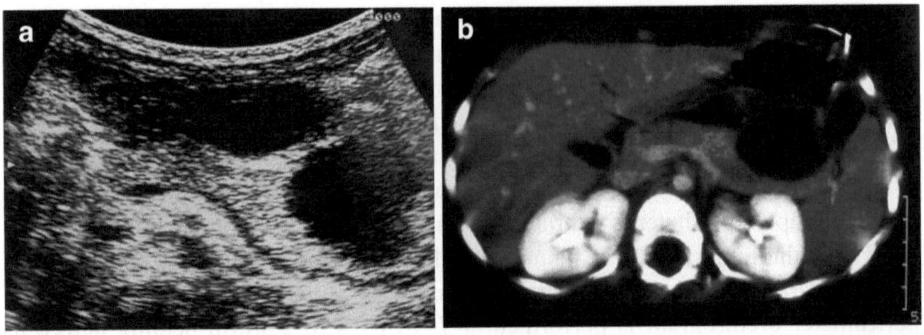

Fig. 4.19 A 6-year-old boy fell on iron stake. Pancreatic isthmus transection with peripancreatic fluid collections. (**a**) US shows pancreatic fluid collections. (**b**) Contrast-enhanced CT demonstrates isthmic transection and confirms the peripancreatic fluid collections

Pancreatic lesions typically appear as total or partial glandular lacerations, in this case with organ separated into two parts [22].

The direct sign of injury is the detection of the tear as a hypoechoic intraparenchymal rhyme; it can be difficult to find on ultrasound exam. Indirect signs can be more easily depictable: focal or diffused pancreatic swelling, unclear organ profiles, focal or diffuse hyperechogenicity of the parenchyma, and presence of fluid periglandular collection (Fig. 4.19a).

There are few reports on the use of CEUS in pancreatic trauma. CEUS can improve the visualization of the rhyme of laceration, which appears strongly hypoechoic compared to the hyperechoic healthy parenchyma.

In the follow-up, US allows to evaluate the possible development of pancreatic pseudocysts and/or abscesses and to monitor its progress [9].

4.8.2 CT

CT exam shows specific and nonspecific signs of pancreatic trauma.

The generic and/or nonspecific signs may include enlargement of the gland, suffuse hypodense undefined profiles as occurs in contusion, thickening of the renal fascia, and hyperdensity of peripancreatic adipose tissue. The presence of hypodense fluid due to lesion of the pancreatic duct or the presence of hyperdense fluid in case of hematoma within the anterior pararenal space and/or periglandular space, although not specific, is a good indicator of pancreatic trauma and can suggest the suspicion of traumatic lesion (Fig. 4.19b). The presence of peritoneal fluid is also a nonspecific sign.

The direct signs are one or more linear hypodense images after intravenous contrast medium crossing the gland more or less deeply, which are an expression of tearing (Fig. 4.20), while separated glandular fragments will appear in the transections (Fig. 4.21).

CT is able to diagnose indirectly the involvement of the pancreatic duct, in relation to the depth of glandular lesions. Further evaluation of the pancreatic duct can be obtained at a deferred time, with MR cholangiopancreatography (MRCP) or percutaneous cholangiography (ERCP), which is more invasive and less fast.

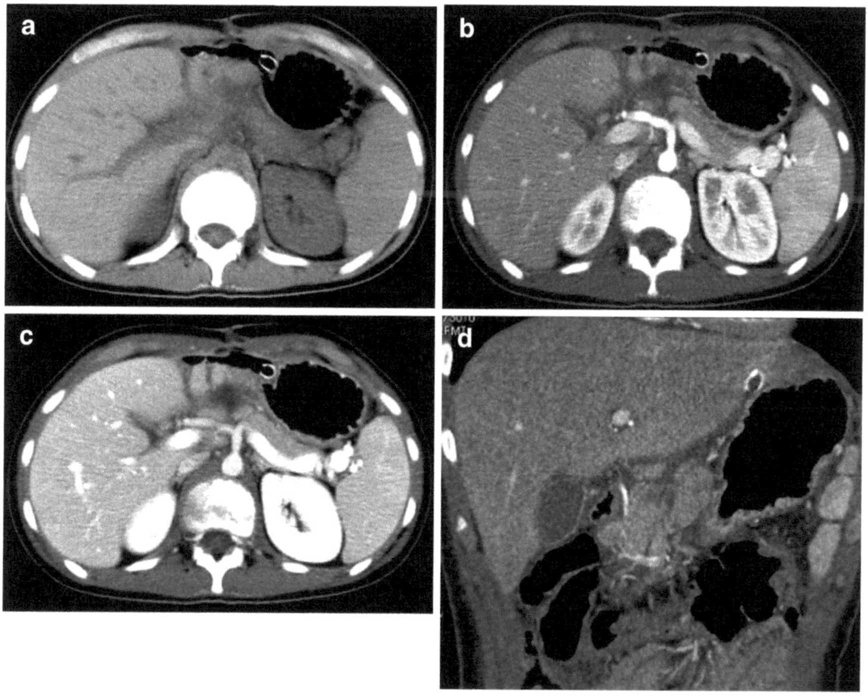

Fig. 4.20 A 15-year-old boy fell during skiing. Pancreatic transection. (**a–d**) Axial and coronal unenhanced and contrast-enhanced CT show pancreatic isthmus transection associated with left hepatic lobe lesion

Periglandular post-traumatic collections, due to duct injury, often evolve into pseudocysts that tend to resolve spontaneously or be subsequently subject to percutaneous drainage or surgery [22].

4.9 Rare Abdominal Injuries

The following injuries are quite rare but not less important.

These are lesions that generally follow a high-energy trauma, their clinical and/or radiological detection is often difficult, and CT is the technique that, generally more than others, can give a significant diagnostic aid.

Bone lesions that are to be found in a major or minor trauma are treated in dedicated chapters [10].

4.9.1 Bowel and Mesentery

Bowel injury is uncommon after blunt trauma in children.

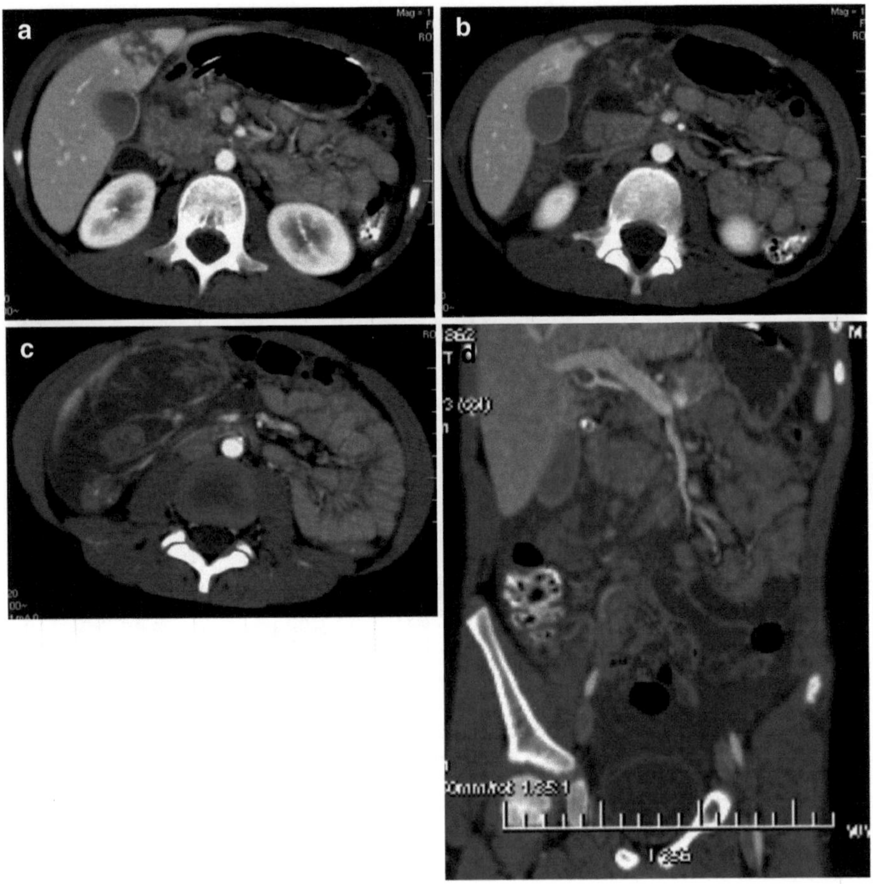

Fig. 4.21 A 16-year-old boy. Motorbike accident. Pancreatic head transection. (**a**–**d**) Axial and coronal contrast-enhanced CT show deep pancreatic tear associated with left hepatic lobe lesion. Huge mesentery root hematoma and relevant amount of hemoperitoneum

Due to the anatomical central position in the abdominal cavity and to the fixation due to the Treitz ligament, lesions of the duodenum and proximal portion of the jejunum are more frequent.

Isolated viscera lesions are usually difficult to diagnose; CT alone cannot be used as a screening tool for hollow viscus injury because the sensitivity and specificity of this technique are approximately 55 and 92 %.

Even clinical signs and symptoms may be absent, minimal, or delayed.

The suspect of hollow viscus injury comes from clinical data, type of trauma, possible presence of superficial abdominal wall bruising, and diagnostic imaging.

US does not usually detect bowel injury; it can demonstrate indirect signs such as free fluid between bowel loops.

As to the abdominal free air presence, depictable through direct abdominal X-ray examination, we must know that the small bowel contains less air than the

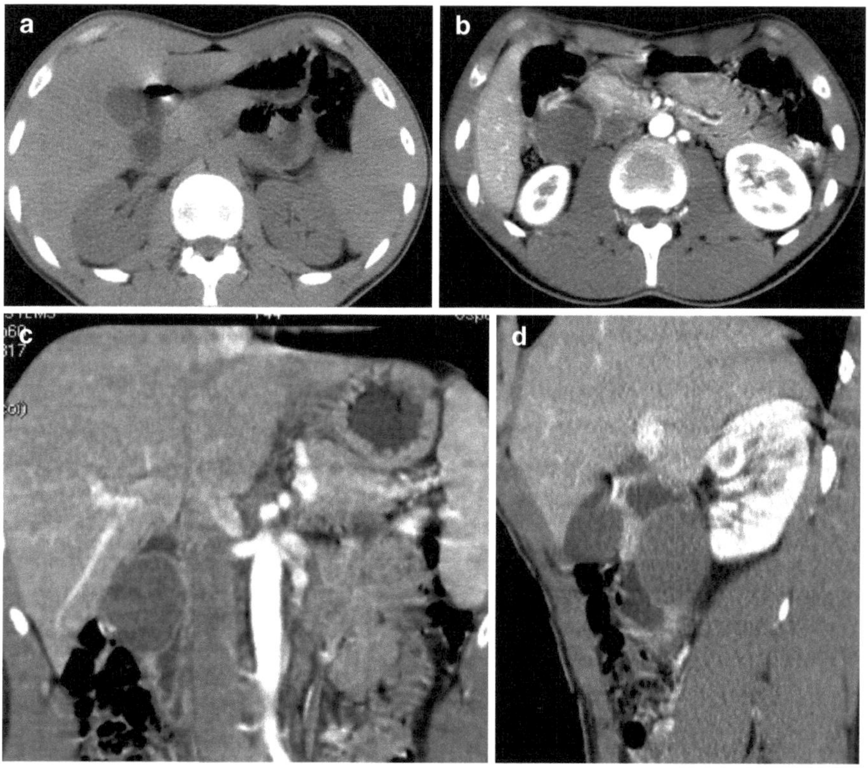

Fig. 4.22 A 17-year-old boy. Car accident. Duodenal hematoma. (**a–d**) Unenhanced and enhanced CT scans show a rounded fluid collection located in the duodenal wall. Note the duodenal lumen compression

large bowel; thus in case of perforation, it will be possible to detect intestinal contents around the injured loop and a small quantity of free air compared to a large bowel perforation.

CT exam shows specific and nonspecific signs.

Specific signs include the tear of the intestinal wall and the presence of free peritoneal or retroperitoneal air which is found by CT exam only approximately in 30–50 % of cases. Bowel wall thickening, usually eccentric, close to the contusive lesion, especially in the duodenum, suggests intramural hematoma (Fig. 4.22). The leakage of the contrast medium through oral administration outside of the intestinal lumen is a highly specific sign; however, it is not very sensitive. Moreover, the use of oral contrast medium is not widely used in the traumatized patient because it takes more time in carrying out the exam.

The complete rupture of the intestine most commonly occurs in the mid to distal part of the small intestine. The most common site is the jejunum.

Nonspecific signs of bowel or mesenteric injury include mesenteric hematoma, which appears as a limited fluid collection of considerable size, which

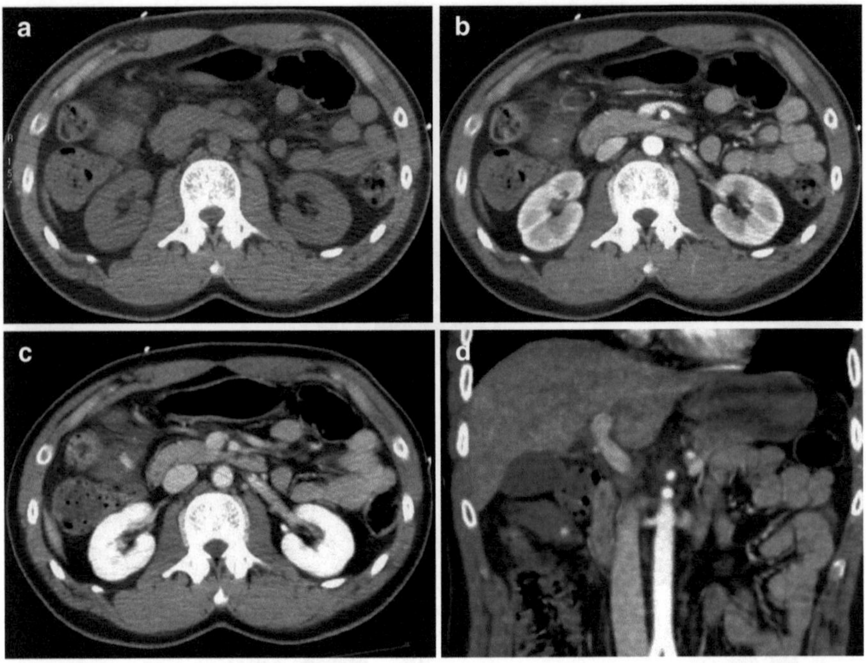

Fig. 4.23 A 17-year-old boy. Microcar accident. Mesenteric hematoma with active bleeding. (**a–c**) Unenhanced and enhanced CT scans show a small amount of fluid in the mesenteric fat. Active bleeding is evident in the arterial phase and increases in the venous phase (**d**) Coronae reconstruction of the same patient

may be seen as active bleeding (Fig. 4.23); free fluid in the abdomen; and "mesenteric stranding" due to mesenteric fat thickening.

4.9.2 Adrenal Glands

Because of the presence of retroperitoneal fat that protects the adrenal glands, traumatic lesions of these glands are very rare in pediatric patients.

The frequency is around 0.15–4 % of blunt abdominal trauma, usually in multiorgan lesions (Fig. 4.24); isolated adrenal injury occurs in around 2–6 % of cases. Traumatic adrenal lesions are more frequent in high-energy trauma with an injury severity score (ISS) >15, associated with other lesions up to 50 %.

Usually traumatic adrenal lesion is unilateral (>90 %) with a considerable prevalence for the right adrenal gland (85–90 %). The prevalence for the right adrenal gland depends on three main causes: abrupt compression between the liver and lumbar vertebral bodies, damage of small vessel due to a deceleration, and the sudden increase of adrenal venous pressure due to the compression of the inferior cava vein (IVC) that highly influences the right adrenal gland because the right adrenal vein drains directly in the IVC. This is the reason why it is influenced more than the left adrenal vein that drains in the left renal vein.

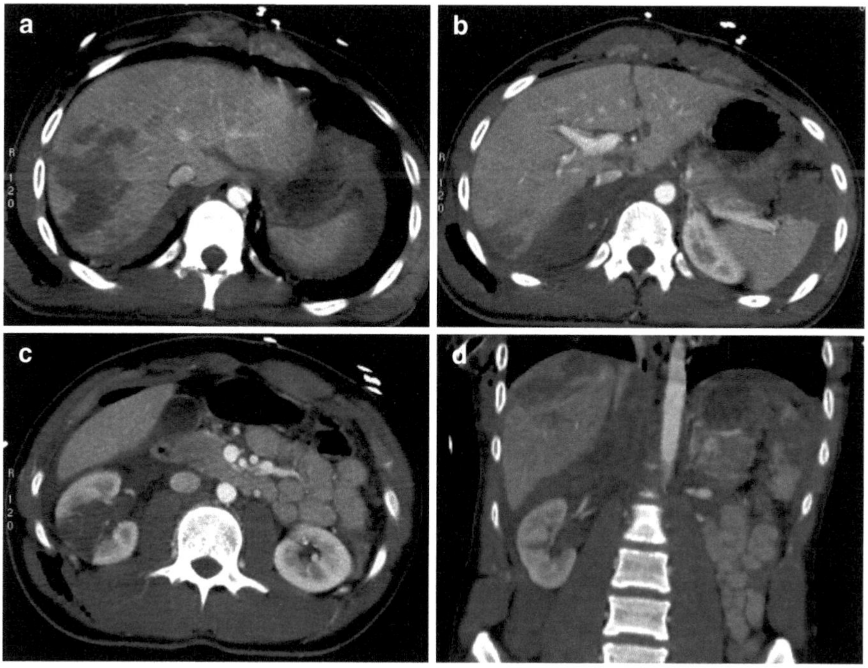

Fig. 4.24 A 16-year-old boy. Motorbike vs. car accident. Multiple organ lesions. (**a–d**) Enhanced CT scans show multiple lesions in the liver, spleen, right kidney, and right adrenal gland. Small focus of active bleeding is shown in the right adrenal space (**b**)

Lesions are usually asymptomatic, so their detection is accidental.

US technique has low sensitivity in detecting traumatic adrenal lesions especially for their association with multiorgan lesions, rib fractures, and pneumothorax [9].

CT is the gold standard exam in detecting traumatic adrenal gland lesions. The main CT details are hematoma around 60–83 %, overall adrenal hemorrhage around 9–43 %, homogeneous swelling of the adrenal gland around 10 %, and adrenal rupture that is very rare.

Furthermore, it is possible to detect associated signs with traumatic lesion such as hemorrhagic suffusion of peri-adrenal fat, retroperitoneal hemorrhage, and active bleeding.

Unrecognized adrenal lesions can cause late hemorrhage and infections. In case of massive hemorrhage, IVC can be compressed causing thrombosis.

Bilateral traumatic adrenal lesions are very rare, less than 1 %; it is still unknown if they can cause severe endocrine anomalies, i.e., acute adrenal failure.

4.9.3 Vessels

Vascular lesions are rare in pediatric trauma. The arteries most frequently involved are the iliolumbar, the superior gluteal, and the internal pudendal because of their proximity to the pelvic bone, the sacroiliac joint, and the inferior ligaments of the pelvis.

Bleeding from the venous network after a pelvic fracture is more frequent than arterial bleeding because the walls of the veins are more fragile than the arteries.

The most frequent pelvic bleeding is due to pelvic bone fracture and/or soft tissue injury.

US exam can only detect fluid collection; in some cases of severe hemorrhage, it is possible to see a fluid corpusculated level in the fluid collection itself, suggesting the hematic component.

CT exam can not only detect vascular injury but also, in many cases, it can differentiate the original bleeding outcome, if it is venous or arterial, and locate the damaged vessel providing all the data needed for a correct arteriographic embolization management.

There are certain CT details such as the promptness in depicting the contrast medium blush in arterial phase and the high blush density that varies according to the aortic density in all examination phases which lead to the arterial nature of the bleeding. The presence of active bleeding near a bone fracture suggests bleeding originating from a bone (Fig. 4.25). The capacity to distinguish the type of bleeding either venous or arterial determines the appropriate management of the patient. An arterial bleeding requires an interventional embolization with a high level of successful outcome, while in case of venous bleeding, it usually requires a nonoperative treatment, which consists, first of all, in restabilizing the normal pelvic volume with wrapping or pelvic fixator to limit the bleeding.

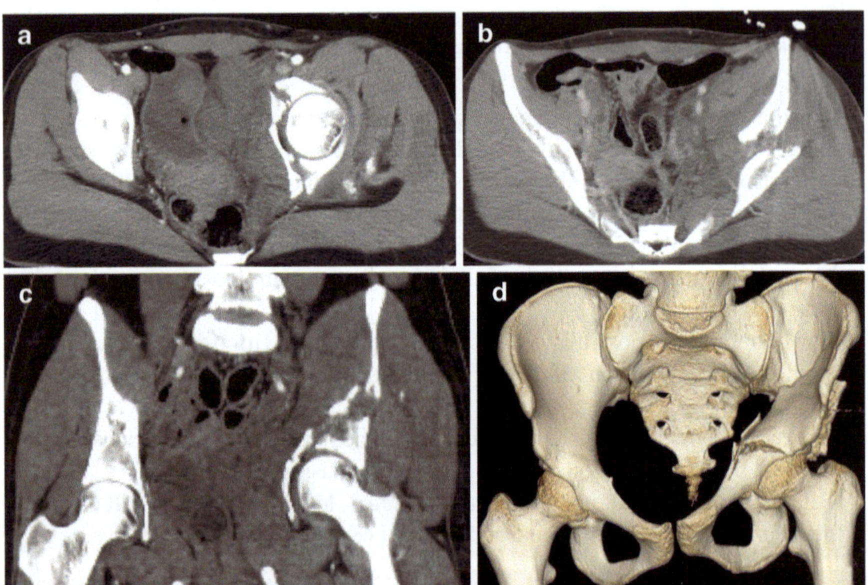

Fig. 4.25 A 16-year-old girl fell from a window. Complex pelvic fracture. (**a**, **b**) Enhanced CT scan in the arterial phase (**a**) shows active bleeding in the left gluteal muscles, while the venous phase (**b**) shows contrast medium leakage in the left obturatory space. (**c**, **d**) Coronal and VR 3D reconstructions show the complex fracture of the pelvic ring, causing instability

Blood may pool in the retroperitoneal space and hemostasis may occur spontaneously in closed fractures, especially if there is no concomitant arterial hemorrhage.

4.9.4 Hypoperfusion Complex

Regardless of the hypovolemic shock causes, the radiologist must recognize and identify a complex set of CT details that are typical expression of severe hypoperfusion and that are suggestive of a transition state between severe but compensated hypovolemia and the decompensated state. In these cases, we have a caliber reduction of the aorta and inferior cava vein and a widespread fluid distention of the intestinal bowel with thickened and irregular enhancement of the bowel wall after contrast medium injection (shock bowel).

There will be a considerable enhancement of the mesentery, kidneys, and adrenal glands, which will then decrease in the pancreatic and spleen parenchyma. It is possible to find periportal low-attenuation zones and peritoneal and retroperitoneal fluid.

The detection of these CT details that suggest hypoperfusion is a predictor of a poor outcome; in fact, the reported mortality rate in children with this set of findings at CT is more than 80 %, and many of these children have severe associated multisystem injury.

References

1. Williams A, Kapila L (2001) Managing an acute abdomen. Curr Pediatr 11:311–316
2. Hynick NH, Brennan M, Schmit P, Noseworthy S, Yanchar NL (2014) Identification of blunt abdominal injuries in children. J Trauma Acute Care Surg 76(N1):95–1000
3. Sivit CJ (2009) Imaging children with abdominal trauma. AJR Am J Roentgenol 192(5):1179–1189
4. Streck CJ Jr, Jewett BM, Wahlquist AH, Gutierrez PS, Russell WS (2012) Evaluation for intra-abdominal injury in children following blunt torso trauma. Can we reduce unnecessary abdominal CT by utilizing a clinical prediction model? J Trauma Acute Care Surg 73(2):371–376
5. Menoch MJ, Hirsh DA, Khan NS, Simon HK, Sturm JJ (2012) Trends in computed tomography utilization in pediatric emergency department. Pediatrics 129(3):e690–e697
6. Pinto F, Miele V, Scaglione M, Pinto A (2013) The use of contrast-enhanced ultrasound in blunt abdominal trauma: advantages and limitations. Acta Radiologica (Epub ahead of print)
7. Miele V, Buffa V, Stasolla A, Regine G, Atzori M, Ialongo P, Adami A (2004) Contrast enhanced ultrasound with second generation contrast agent in traumatic liver lesions. Radiol Med 107:82–91
8. Cagini L, Gravante S, Malaspina M, Cesarano E, Giganti M, Rebornato A, Fonio P, Scialpi M (2013) Contrast enhanced ultrasound (CEUS) in blunt abdominal trauma. Crit Ultrasound J 5(Suppl 1):1–7
9. Valentino M, De Luca C, Galloni SS, Branchini M, Modolon C, Pavlica P, Barozzi L (2010) Contrast Enhanced US evaluation in patients with blunt abdominal trauma. J Ultrasound 13:22–27
10. Cronan JJ, Kane NM, De Luca F (1988) Pediatric abdominal trauma: evaluation by computed tomography. Pediatrics 82(1):11–15

11. Patrick DA, Bensard DD, Moore EE, Terry SJ, Karree FM (1998) Ultrasound is an effective triage tool to evaluate blunt abdominal trauma in the pediatric population. J Trauma 45(1):57–63
12. Tseng YC, Lee MS, Chang YJ, Wu HP (2008) Acute abdomen in pediatric patient admitted to the Pediatric Emergency Department. Pediatr Neonatol 49(4):126–134
13. Bulas DI, Eichelberger MR, Sivit CJ, Wright CJ, Gotschall CS (1993) Hepatic injury from blunt trauma in children: follow-up evaluation with CT. AJR Am J Roentgenol 160:347–351
14. Yi IK, Miao FL, Wong J, Narasimhan KL, Lo RH, Yee L, Stringer DA, Sundfor AJ (2010) Prophylactic embolization of hepatic artery pseudoaneurysm after blunt abdominal trauma in a child. J Pediatr Surg 45:837–839
15. Shanmuganathan K, Mirvis SE, Boyd-Kranis R, Takada T, Scalea TM (2000) Nonsurgical management of blunt splenic injury: use of CT criteria to select patients for splenic arteriography and potential endovascular therapy. Emerg Radiol 1:75–82
16. Fick AEA, Raychaudhuri P, Bear J, Roy G, Balogh Z, Kumar R (2011) Factors predicting need for splenectomy in children with blunt splenic trauma. ANZ J Surg 81:717–719
17. Lippert SJ, Hartin CW Jr, Ozgediz DE, Glick PL, Caty MG, Flynn WJ, Bass KD (2013) Splenic conservation: variation between pediatric and adult trauma centers. J Surg Res 182(1):17–20
18. Brennan TV, Lipshutz GS, Posselt AM, Horn JK (2003) Congenital cleft spleen with CT scan appearance of high-grade splenic laceration after blunt abdominal trauma. J Emerg Med 2:139–142
19. St Peter SD, Aguayo P, Juang D, Sharp SW, Snyder CL, Holcomb GW 3rd, Ostlie DJ (2013) Follow up of prospective validation of an abbreviated bed rest protocol in the management of blunt spleen and liver injury in children. J Pediatr Surg 48:2437–2441
20. Graziano KD, Juang D, Notrica D, Grandsoult VL, Acosta J, Sharp SW, Murphy JP, St. Peter SD (2014) Prospective observational study with an abbreviated protocol in the management of blunt renal injury in children. J Pediatr Surg 49:198–201
21. Regine G, Atzori M, Miele V, Buffa V, Galluzzo M, Luzietti M, Adami L (2007) Second-generation sonographic contrast agents in the evaluation of renal trauma. Radiol Med 112:581–587
22. Miele V, Patti G, Galluzzo M, Bibbolino C, Adami L (1998) Isolated pancreatic rupture caused by abdominal blunt trauma in a child. Study with spiral computerized tomography. Radiol Med 96:256–258
23. Iqbal CW, St. Peter SD, Tsao K, Cullinane DC, Gourlay DM, Ponsky TA, Wlkan ML, Adibe OO (2014) Operative vs non operative management for blunt pancreatic transection in children: multi institutional outcomes. J Am Coll Surg 218:157–162

Imaging Bone Injuries with Plain Film X-Ray

5

Michele Tonerini, Francesco Ruschi, Alessandra Scionti, and Umberto Tani

5.1 Introduction

Musculoskeletal injuries are common in children and adolescents and their incidence had been increasing in the past 20 years because of the widespread use of motorized and high-speed wheeled vehicles [1, 2]. Nowadays they account for 15–20 % of causes of admission in the emergency department, but thanks to the unique properties of immature bone, in most cases the anatomical damage has a modest extension and a great healing capacity after an adequate treatment. Nevertheless, in order to avoid a deformity, the diagnosis and the therapy must be prompt, especially when the lesion involves the physis. Young boys are affected more than girls and elbow and wrist fractures are usually the most frequent ones. However carpal fractures are rare in children and, when they occur, often involve the scaphoid [3, 4]. Children often are difficult to examine, and so, physical examination may be somewhat short, negative, or even obtuse. Infants often cry at the sight of an intruding physician, and so the physical examination may be very difficult. At this point, the physician usually proceeds to the laboratory and imaging investigation. Both sources of information are important, but imaging usually is the most important part of this investigative cohort [5, 6].

M. Tonerini (✉)
Department of Emergency Radiology, Cisanello Hospital, Pisa, Italy
e-mail: m.tonerini@tiscali.it

F. Ruschi • A. Scionti • U. Tani
Department of Diagnostic Imaging, Cisanello Hospital, Pisa, Italy
e-mail: e-mail: francescoruschi@gmail.com, alessandra86sc@gmail.com, umbetani@gmail.com

V. Miele, M. Trinci (eds.), *Imaging Trauma and Polytrauma in Pediatric Patients*,
DOI 10.1007/978-3-319-08524-1_5

5.2 Bone Development and Anatomy

The histological structure and the biomechanics of the pediatric bone are different from those of the adult, determining peculiar musculoskeletal injuries, healing mechanisms, and a different management [7–9]. Skeletal injuries in children vary according to the age in relation to the anatomical, biomechanical, and physiological features typical of the maturing skeleton influenced by endocrine factors such as growth hormone (GH), thyroxine, estrogen, and testosterone. The pediatric bone is less dense, more porous, and penetrated throughout by capillary channels, with respect to the adult one. The lower bending strength and elasticity of the immature skeleton determine more strain and allow for greater energy absorption before failure. At the same time, its higher sponginess prevents propagation of fractures and reduces the incidence of comminuted forms. The children's periosteum is stronger and thicker than the adult one, both functioning in reduction and maintenance of fracture alignment. Moreover, thanks to its rich vascularization, it plays an important role in a faster bone healing [10, 11]. Another important difference between the pediatric and the adult skeleton relies on the cartilaginous growth plate which is able to absorb the traumatic energy prior to get fractured. On the other side it represents a locus of minor resistance, because the higher resistance and flexibility of tendons and ligaments compared to the physis may lead to its disruption or avulsion. The changes during puberty, such as the increase of muscle strength and the rapid growth, together with the peculiar pediatric bone structure, explain why the plate avulsion fracture is more common in children [12, 13]. Its late diagnosis and treatment may determine abnormalities in skeletal maturation or growth arrest and so a paramount attention must be posed in the clinical suspicion of a physeal injury. The two physiological mechanisms of bone production and development are endochondral (long bones) and intramembranous ossification (flat bones). In the long bones of the immature skeleton, we can describe four main regions: diaphysis, metaphysis, epiphysis, and physis [12, 14]. The *diaphysis* is the elongated shaft characterized by variably mature lamellar bone covered by thick periosteum. The *metaphysis* is the wide area below the physis and closest to the diaphysis and it is constituted by a spongy, inner substance covered by thin laminar cortical bone. At each extremity of the bone, there is the *epiphysis*, which contains the ossifying center and the cartilage-covered articular portion. The growth plate, or *physis*, lies between the epiphysis and the metaphysis; it is represented by cartilage cells that create solid bone with growth and it is responsible for the majority of longitudinal bone development. It is very important to preserve its integrity in order to avoid abnormalities of the skeletal growth. Another key component is the *periosteum*, which is a circumferential, thick, nutrient layer, which serves a major role in healing the outer layer of bone [1, 11, 15].

5.3 Pediatric Fracture Patterns

The mechanism of the fractures varies according to children's age [2, 3, 7, 10, 13]. Younger kids are more likely to sustain a fracture while playing and falling on an outstretched arm, while the older ones tend to injure themselves while playing sports

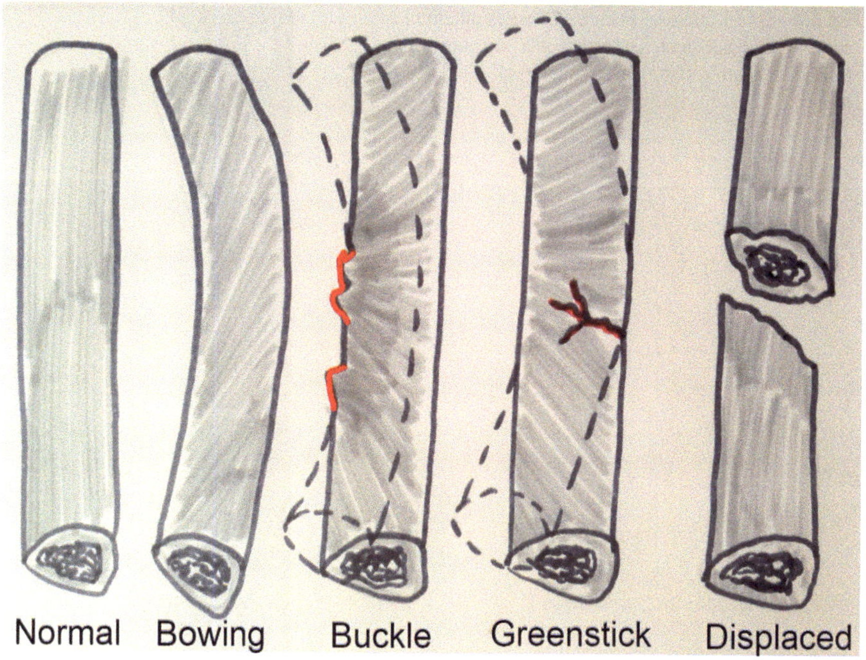

Fig. 5.1 A drawing representing the different fracture patterns in pediatric age

and riding bicycles and in motor vehicle accidents. It must be kept in mind that the child's ligaments are stronger than those of an adult; consequently the traumatic forces, which could determine a sprain in an older individual, will be transmitted to the bone and cause a fracture in a child. Caution should therefore be exercised when assessing a young child diagnosed with a sprain. These differences between children and adults skeleton result in different fracture patterns [16–19], which in the pediatric age are represented by complete fractures, plastic deformations, buckled fractures, greenstick fractures, apophyseal injuries, and physeal fractures (Fig. 5.1).

A *complete fracture* is a break that runs the entire width of a bone and it is classified as spiral, transverse, or oblique, depending on the direction of the fracture line [2, 5]. *Spiral fractures* are usually caused by a rotational, low-velocity force (Fig. 5.2). An intact periosteal hinge enables the orthopedic surgeon to reduce the fracture by reversing the rotational injury [1, 8]. *Oblique fractures* occur diagonally across the diaphyseal bone and they are unstable; therefore an alignment is necessary (Fig. 5.3). A fracture reduction is attempted by immobilizing the extremity while applying traction [3]. *Transverse fractures* are determined by a three-point bending force and usually they are easily reduced by using the intact periosteal layer from the concave side of the fracture force (Fig. 5.4). Many of them involve the upper extremities [10, 11] and the clavicle is a typical example (Fig. 5.5). In most cases, fracture of the clavicle concerns the outer third and it is the consequence of a direct blow to the acromion which causes the epiphysis (firmly anchored by the strong acromioclavicular ligaments) to separate from the growth plate and ride upward. Complete mid-shaft clavicular fractures are rare and the medial fragment is

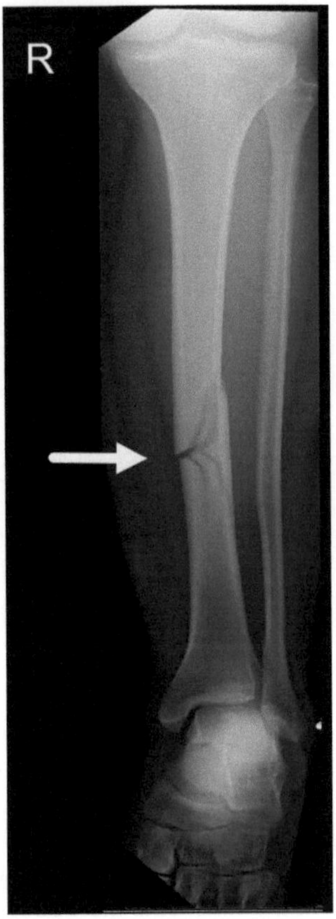

Fig. 5.2 Spiral fracture. Female, 14 years old, after a motor vehicle accident. The anterior X-ray shows a spiral displaced fracture of the diaphyseal tibial shaft (*arrow*)

usually elevated by the sternocleidomastoid muscle, so that it can be easily displayed on the plain films [12]. The fracture of the distal humerus is more common in children than in adults, but the diagnosis may be difficult owing to the numerous ossification centers. In 60 % of cases, the fracture concerns the supracondylar region and it is crucial to promptly immobilize the arm in order to avoid a neurovascular injury (Fig. 5.6). Lateral condyle and medial epicondyle fractures have a lower incidence (respectively, 15 and 10 %) and the consequence of a delayed diagnosis is severe, since the former has a high potential for nonunion and the latter may be frequently associated with an ulnar nerve injury. The *fat pad sign* [20, 21] may be the radiological manifestation of an occult fracture in the elbow and it is determined by the distention of a structurally intact joint capsule. Three small masses of fat rest in the radial, coronoid, and olecranon fossae and are enveloped by the fibers of the joint capsule, which separate the fat pads from the synovial lining, making them intracapsular and extrasynovial in location. When there is a joint distention, the anterior fat pad is displaced anteriorly and superiorly and the posterior fat pad is displaced posteriorly and superiorly. The previously invisible posterior fat pad becomes visible on the lateral radiograph of the elbow held in 90° of flexion.

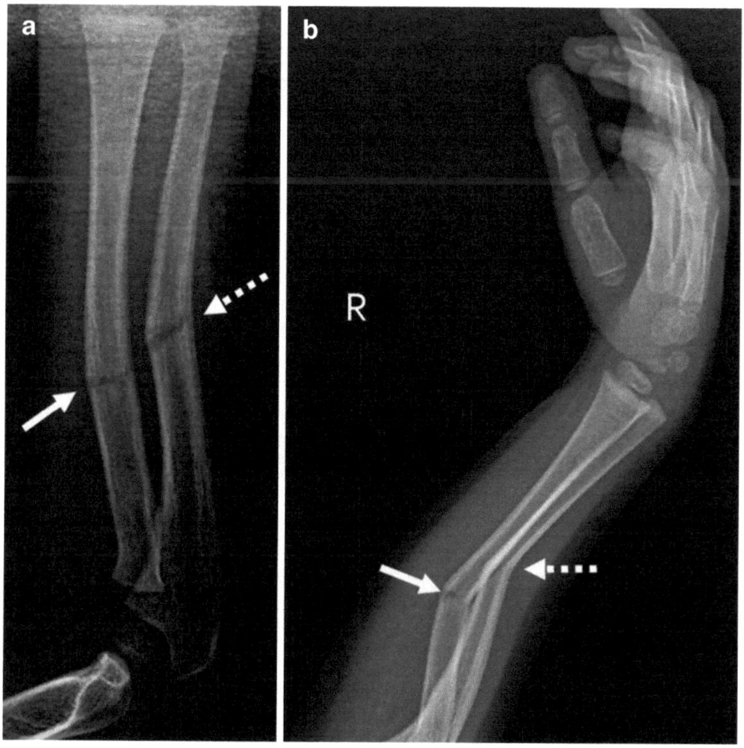

Fig. 5.3 Oblique and transverse fractures. Female, 3 years old, fallen accidentally downward a table. The anterior (**a**) and the lateral (**b**) plain films display an oblique fracture of the ulnar shaft (*dashed arrow*) and a transverse fracture of the radial diaphysis (*arrow*), both angulated

However, it must be remembered that not only hemarthrosis or joint effusion due to trauma but also infections, inflammations, or neoplasms can distend the joint capsule and displace the fat pads [21]. Proximal humeral fractures are rare (about 1 % of all the pediatric fractures) and they may be determined by an underlying pathology, such as a bone cyst or a benign tumor (Fig. 5.7). Since the proximal humerus provides for the majority of the longitudinal growth of this bone and has therefore a high remodeling potential, the surgical treatment is not required, and up until the age of 5, a slight degree of fragment angulation is tolerable for a good healing [22, 23]. Forearm fractures are most frequent in children and they are usually associated fractures, meaning that both the radius and the ulna (Figs. 5.4 and 5.5) or the distal radioulnar joint is involved at the same time [11, 23]. In children, the most common forearm fractures concern the distal region of the radius and they are similar to the adult ones both for features and traumatic mechanism (typical are Colles' fracture and Smith's fracture). The only difference with elderly patients consists in the treatment, as in children these fractures usually do not involve the joint and the bones have a high remodeling potential so major angulations may be tolerable [24, 25]. Injuries of the proximal region of the radius usually involve the "neck" (Fig. 5.8)

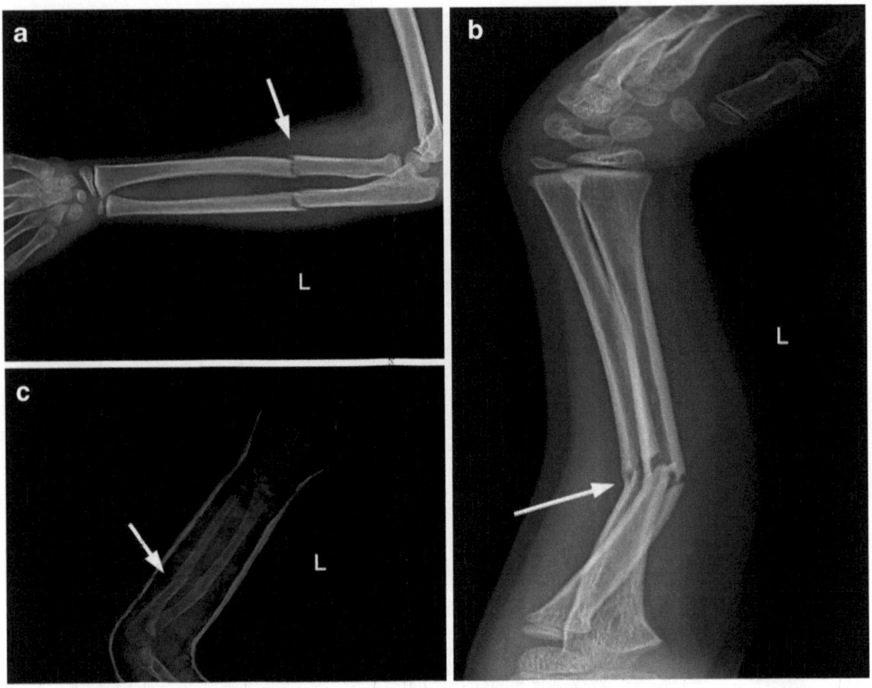

Fig. 5.4 Transverse, displaced fractures. Male, 7 years old, fallen from bicycle with the outstretched forearm. X-rays show a transverse, displaced fracture of both radial and ulnar shaft (*arrows*) in the anterior (**a**) and in the lateral plain film (**b**) and the following reduction in cast (**c**)

Fig. 5.5 Clavicular fracture. Male, 3 years old, fallen from a cockhorse. In the anterior X-ray, there is an undisplaced transverse fracture of the right clavicular shaft (*arrow*)

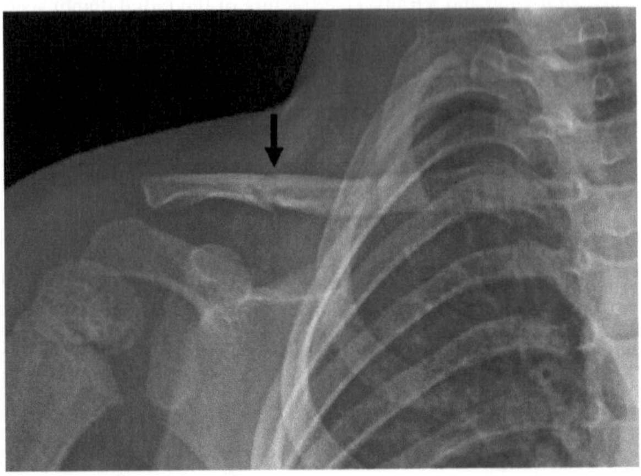

because the epiphysis is cartilaginous until the age of 3–6 and it is therefore more resistant to trauma forces. The mechanism is a fall with an open hand on an outstretched and externally rotated arm. Radial fractures may be classified according to the Judet classification [26, 27] which is based on the angulation between the

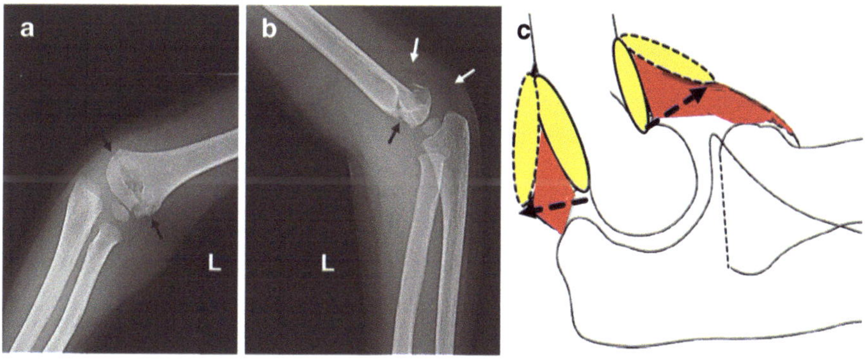

Fig. 5.6 Supracondylar humeral fracture. Female, 33 months old. Slipped while running. The anterior (**a**) and the lateral (**b**) plain films display a slightly displaced supracondylar humeral fracture (*black arrows*) and the posterior fat pad sign (*white arrows*). In (**c**) a schematic drawing of the anatomic explanation of the fat pad sign: when there is a joint distention, the anterior fat pad is displaced anteriorly and superiorly (*dashed arrow* on the right) and the posterior fat pad is displaced posteriorly and superiorly (*dashed arrow* on the left)

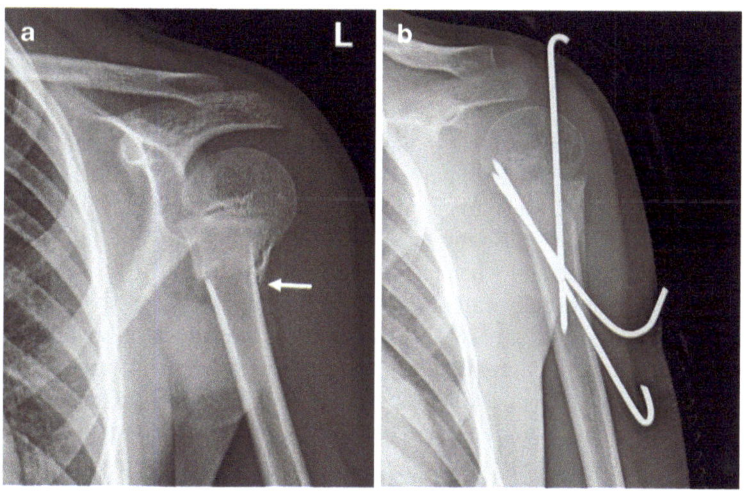

Fig. 5.7 Proximal humeral fracture. Female, 8 years old. Fallen during sport activity. The anterior plain films show a complete, displaced fracture of the proximal left humeral metaphysis (*arrow* in **a**) treated with surgical repair (**b**)

fragments into four grades of severity (Fig. 5.9). A particular kind of associated injury of the radius and ulna is the Monteggia fracture that involves the proximal region of the ulna and is associated with the anterior dislocation of the proximal radius [1, 11]. Fractures of the lower extremities in children are rarer than in adults due to the thick periosteum and the greater content in cartilage that allows a traumatic energy absorption. Pelvic, sacrum, and femoral injuries are all uncommon and they account for 2–8 % of all pediatric fractures. Tibial traumas are slightly

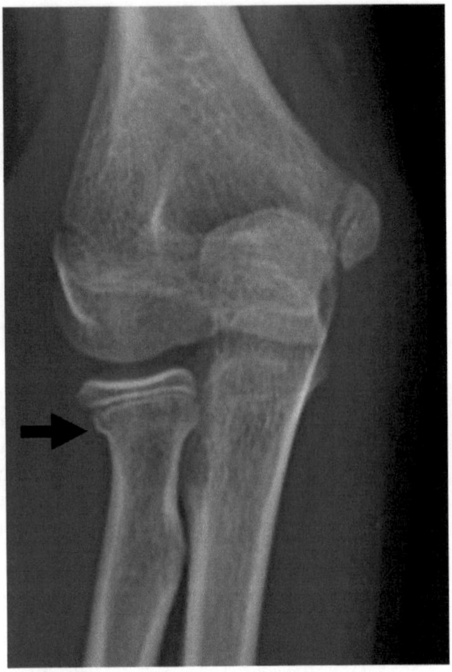

Fig. 5.8 Radial neck fracture. Male, 17 years old, fallen with an open hand on the outstretched and externally rotated arm. The anterior radiograph reveals an undisplaced fracture of the metaphyseal portion of the radial neck (*arrow*)

more frequent, usually happen in young boys from 8 to 13 years old, and are caused by a fall on an outstretched and internally rotated leg, as in a bicycle fall. The same mechanism in adults may lead to an injury to the anterior "cruciate" ligament while in younger patients may cause the fracture of the tibial spine. Injuries of the tibial shaft are frequent especially when infant begins to walk (from 10 months to 3 years old) and so they are usually called *toddler's* fractures (Fig. 5.10). They are often closed and incomplete [4, 11, 28, 29]. A plastic deformation (or bowing fracture) occurs when a traumatic force produces microscopic failure on the tensile (convex) side of a long bone which does not propagate to the concave side. Consequently the shaft is angulated beyond its elastic limit, resulting in a persistent deformation (Fig. 5.11). The cortex, under the periosteum, has a lower mineral content than the adult one and an increased porosity, due to larger and more abundant Haversian canals; this allows the bone to bent, buckle, or bow but not to break when compressed [13, 15]. In this particular type of injury, there is not an evident fracture line but numerous microfractures on the concave surface of the diaphysis with an intact cortex on the convex side. It is most common in the forearm, especially in the ulna, associated with fracture of the radius, but occasionally it can involve the fibula, the tibia, and the clavicle. Plastic deformation can occur isolated but more commonly it happens together with a fracture of the adjacent bone, meaning that the presence of a fracture in a pediatric skeletal segment should suggest the radiologist to look for deformation in the other one. Sometimes there is a detachment of the periosteal surface with a hematoma. The diagnosis of a bending fracture, often difficult, may be easier using the comparative plain film views [30]. A plastic deformation of the

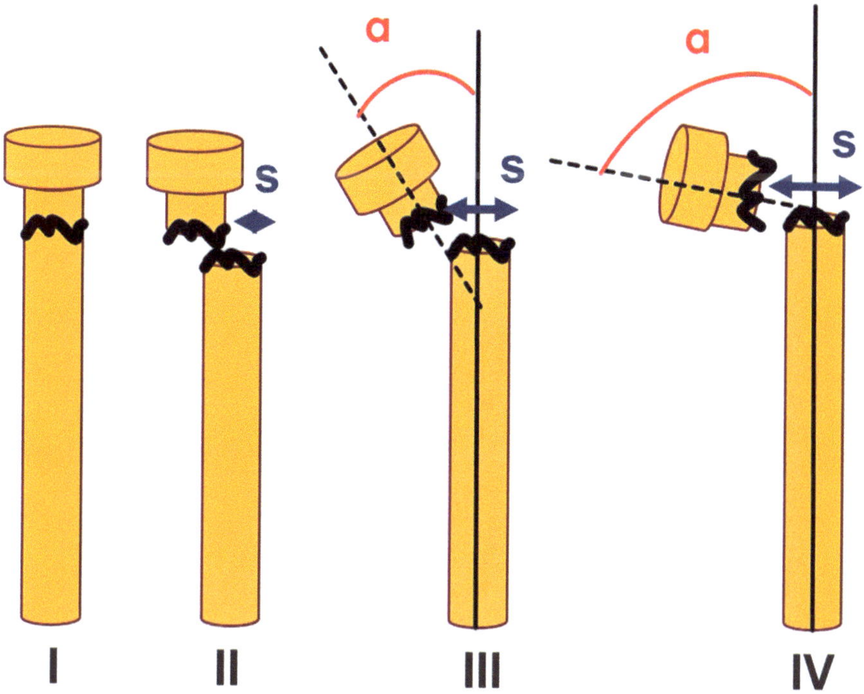

Fig. 5.9 Diagram illustrating the classification of fractures of the radial neck by Judet et al.: grade I, undisplaced fracture; grade II, $\alpha < 30°$ (angulation of radial neck), $S < 1/2$ diameter of radial shaft (translation <50 %); grade III, $\alpha = 30°$ to $60°$, $S < 1/1$ diameter of radial shaft (translation <100 %); grade IV, $\alpha = 60°$ to $90°$, $S > 1/1$ diameter of radial shaft (translation >100 %)

clavicle, consequent to a fall on an outstretched hand or a direct blow to the shoulder, is especially easy to be missed, even with the comparative views, which will show a mild asymmetry of the shafts. A bowing fracture sometimes must be straightened or broken to effect reduction [17, 20, 22]. Buckle fracture (or torus fracture) is the result of a compression failure of bone that usually occurs at the junction of the metaphysis and the diaphysis, where the cortical is less thick, owing to the prevalence of the spongious bone (Fig. 5.12). The term "torus" comes from the Latin word which means swelling which refers to the enlargement that separates the capitellum from the body of the classical column and it is due to the characteristic angulation of the cortex following a pure axial force applied on a hyperextended or hyperflexed bone segment. It is the most common fracture in children and it is easily missed [1, 3], because the only radiological sign is an angled buckle caused by the trabecular compression, while the periosteal and cortical layers on the other side are intact (Fig. 5.13). A typical traumatic mechanism is a fall over an overextended limb with bending of the bone and compression on the concave side: this occurs most commonly at the distal radius following a fall on an outstretched arm. Other common sites for torus fractures are the wrist (Fig. 5.14), the elbow, and the ankle [30]. Buckle (torus) fractures are common in infants and children and generally occur

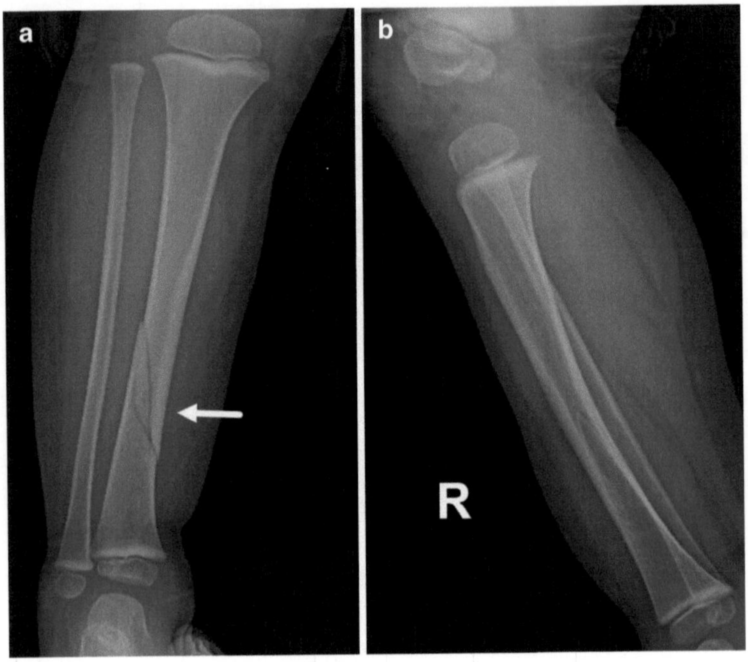

Fig. 5.10 Toddler's fracture. Male, 3 years old. The spiral fracture of the third distal of the right tibial shaft (*arrow*) is easily displayed in the anterior plain film (**a**) but it is very difficult to be appreciated in the lateral radiograph (**b**)

through the metaphyses of long bones (Fig. 5.15). There are two different types of buckle fractures [31]: the classic form and the angled form (Fig. 5.16). The classic form results from axial loading of the long bone with resultant compression of the bone and buckling of the trabeculae along the fracture line. This leads to outward, decompressive, unilateral, or bilateral bulging of the cortex at either end of the fracture line. In the angled form, however, only angulation of the cortex is seen and it usually results from initial axial loading on a long bone but, in addition, associated forces in varus, valgus, hyperextension, or hyperflexion. Depending on which of these is present, the fracture will be seen on the dorsal, ventral, medial, or lateral aspect of the involved long bone [28, 30, 31]. Even if an underlying trabecular compressive fracture is always present in these patients, they usually are not appreciable at the initial time of injury. However, substantiating sclerosis along the fracture zone attests to their presence. Angled buckle fractures usually are isolated, subtle, and easily overlooked. However, once one becomes familiar with their appearance and where they tend to occur, one can diagnose them with more certainty, especially if comparative views are utilized. Soft tissue changes (soft tissue swelling and fat pad obliteration or displacement) also are important as they serve to focus one's attention on the site of injury and so cause one to look more closely for a possible fracture. Buckle fractures are inherently stable and usually heal in 3–4 weeks with simple immobilization [17, 20, 23]. Greenstick fracture is an incomplete fracture of

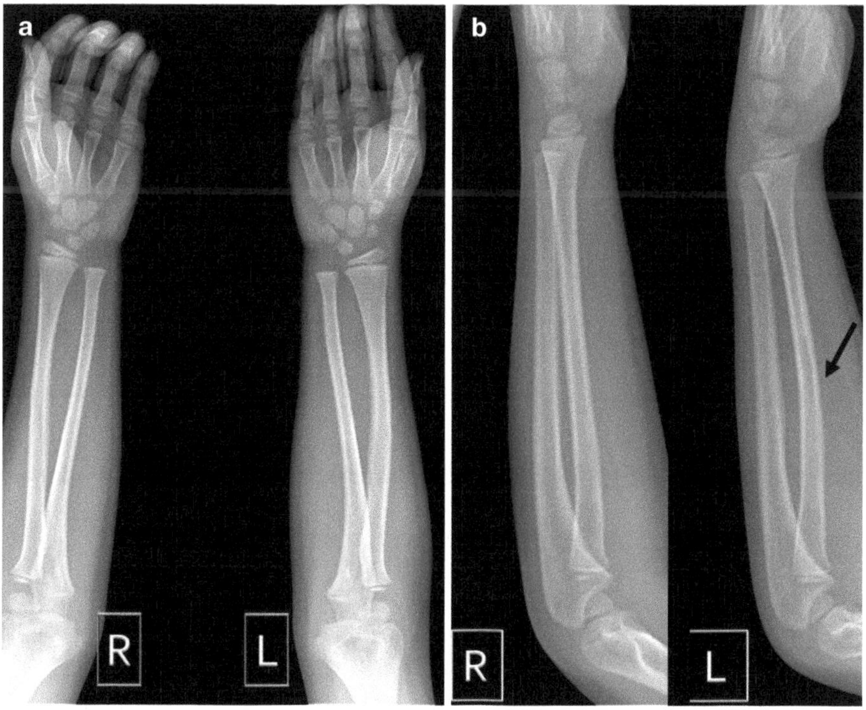

Fig. 5.11 Plastic deformation. Male, 5 years old, fallen from a table on the overstretched arm. A comparative X-ray study of the forearms was performed in anterior (**a**) and lateral projection (**b**). There is a plastic deformation (bowing fracture) of the left radial shaft which is clearly appreciable only in the lateral plain film (**b**, *arrow*). This case underlines the importance of the two orthogonal plain films in the evaluation of pediatric skeletal injuries

the metaphysis or diaphysis of the long bones (Fig. 5.17). The name "greenstick" comes from the fracture's similarity with green, fresh wood which also breaks on the convex side when bent, without a complete line. It occurs when the traumatic force (an angulated longitudinal force or perpendicular force, like a direct blow) causes a disruption of the convex surface of the shaft, but it is not enough to break it completely into separate pieces [3]. It is sometimes associated with plastic deformation on the opposite side. The typical site is the diaphysis or the metaphysis of the wrist. This fracture usually requires immobilization, but if the shaft undergoes a plastic deformation, it is necessary to break the skeletal segment on the concave side to restore a normal alignment, as the plastic deformation recoils the bone back to the deformed position. While the physes are the primary ossification centers (located at the ends of the long bones) and are responsible for longitudinal bone growth, the apophyses are the secondary centers of ossification (found where major tendons attach to bone) and provide contour and shape to growing bones without adding length. Since cartilage is less resistant to tensile forces than bones, ligaments, and muscle-tendon units, these growth centers are the weakest links in the

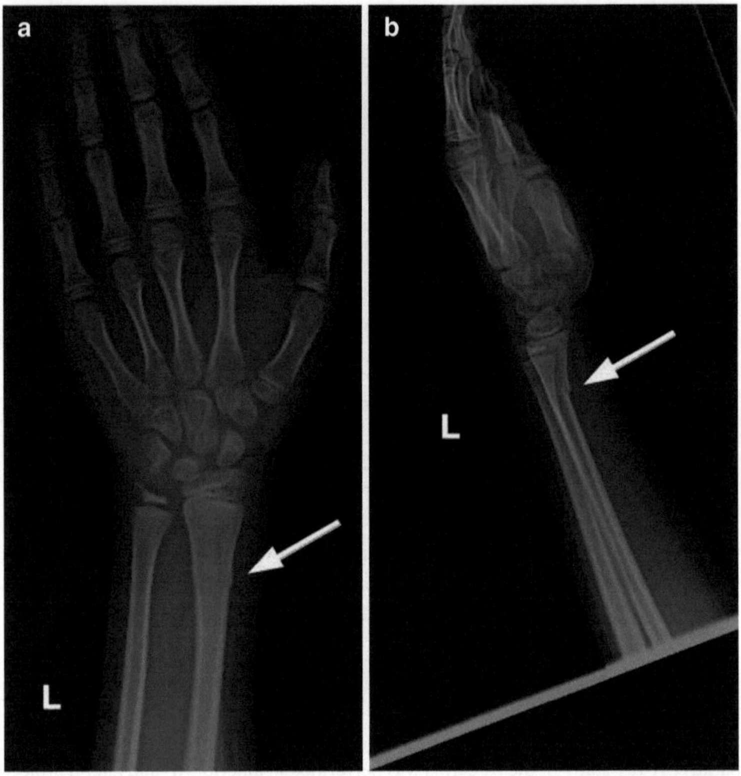

Fig. 5.12 Buckle fracture. Male, 10 years old, fallen while playing soccer. The anterior (**a**) and lateral (**b**) plain films show a classic type buckle fracture of the third distal of the left radial diaphysis (*arrow*)

musculoskeletal chain. The same injury mechanisms that cause muscle strains and tendonitis in adults result in growth center injuries in children and teens [32, 33]. *Apophyseal injuries* usually occur in adolescents playing sports and are often described on the hip bones (ischial tuberosity, iliac spine, pubic ramus, iliac crest, greater and lesser trochanter), the knee (inferior pole of the patella and anterior tibial tubercle), and the spine (secondary ossifying site of the vertebral soma) owing to the greater number of growing plates of these bone districts [34, 35]. Usually they can be diagnosed by history and physical examination and radiographs are needed to rule out fractures or bone lesions, when the presentation is less clear. Utrasonography (US) and magnetic resonance imaging (MRI) play a major role in the definition of the type of lesion and in the depiction of the ligamentous and tendinous compartment [36] (Fig. 5.18). Physeal fractures are those involving the growth plate that is the weakest area in children's bone and they represent approximately 15 % of all fractures in children. The distal radial physis is the most frequently injured one. Most physeal injuries heal within 3 weeks, and, as a consequence, there is a limited window of time for reduction of deformity. The damage to

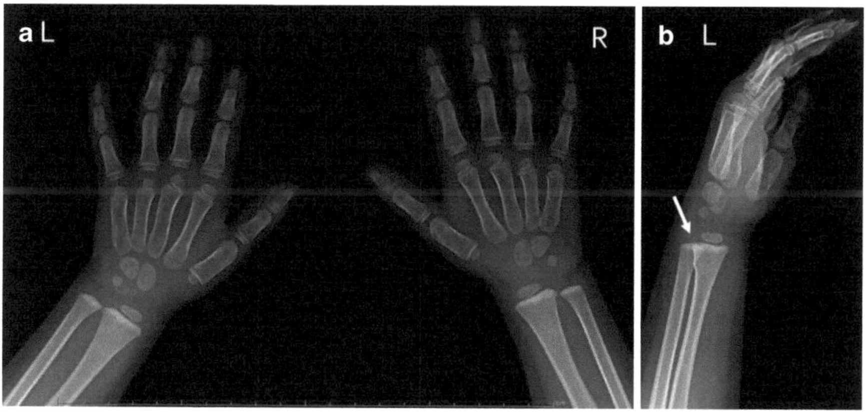

Fig. 5.13 Buckle fracture. Female, 3 years old, fallen downward from a slide on the overstretched arm. The left radial metaphyseal buckle fracture (*arrow*) is clearly appreciable only in the lateral plain film (**b**), while it is difficult to be identified in the comparative anterior plain film (**a**) because the injury involves exclusively the dorsal profile of the radial metaphysis

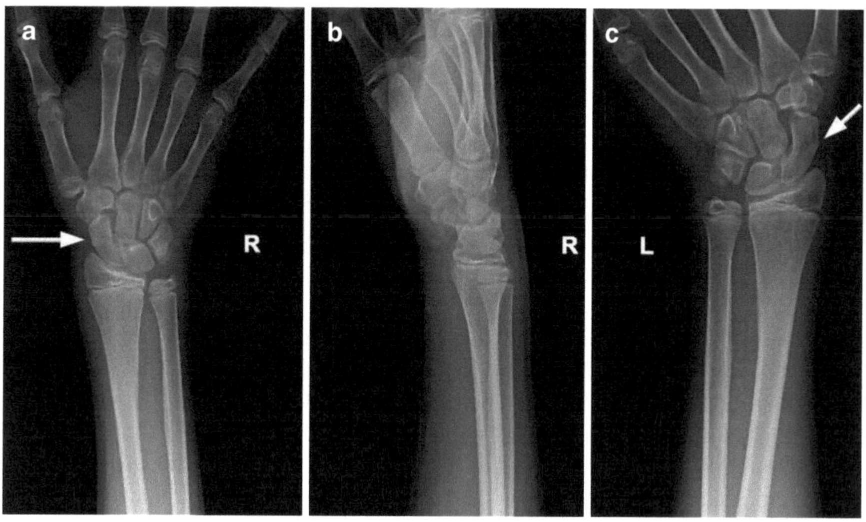

Fig. 5.14 Buckle fracture. Male, 13 year old, fallen on the right overstretched arm while walking on a wet board. The anterior plain film (**a**) of the right wrist shows a buckle fracture of the cortical bone of the scaphoid (*arrow*). This lesion cannot be clearly identified in the lateral view (**b**). The comparative anterior plain film (**c**) shows a normal scaphoid bone on the left side (*arrow*)

growth plate may result in progressive angular deformity, limb-length discrepancy, or joint incongruity [18]. The Salter-Harris (S-H) classification continues to be the most commonly used system for characterizing them and it consists of five types of injuries, which are listed by their location (Fig. 5.19). This classification system is important to plan a correct treatment and so to decrease the risk of growth disturbances and angular deformities [33, 37], as children's bones heal faster than adult

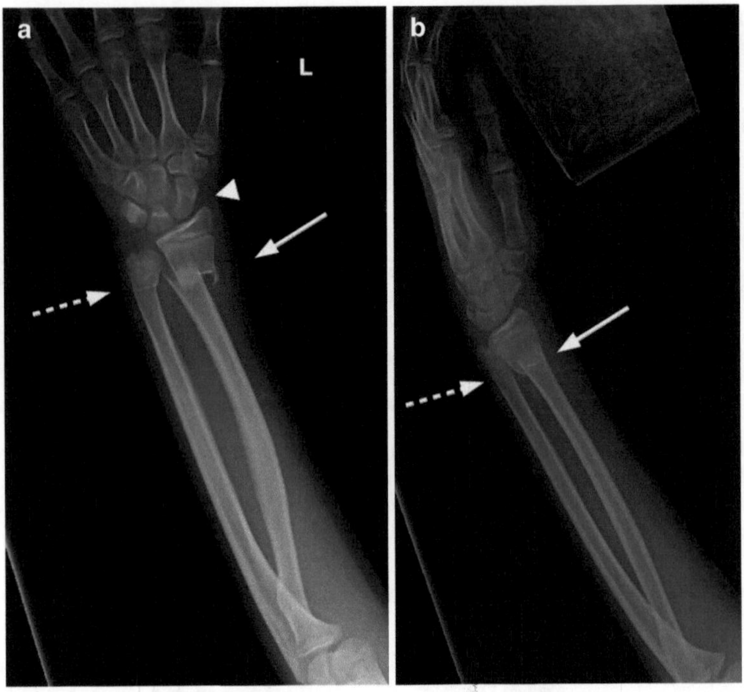

Fig. 5.15 Combined fractures. Male, 14 years old, injured at the left forearm, after a motor vehicle collision. The anterior (**a**) and the lateral (**b**) plain films show a transversal, displaced fracture of the distal radial metaphysis (*arrow*), a buckle fracture of the distal ulnar metaphysis (*dashed arrow*), and a scaphoid buckle injury (*arrowhead*)

ones due to their stronger periosteum. The S-H system divides the fractures into five categories [9, 24] depending upon the type of damage to the growth plate, and a mnemonic way to remember them is the acronym SALTR (slip of physis, type 1; above than physis, type 2; lower than physis, type 3; through the physis, type 4; rammed physis, type 5). *Type I S-H* fractures (Fig. 5.20) occur when there is a complete separation of the entire physis (usually through areas of hypertrophic and degenerating cartilage cell columns) and the surrounding bone is not involved. Plain X-film appears normal because the physis is radiolucent; reduction and immobilization are needed because healing is rapid and the risk of complications after immobilization is extremely low [33]. *Type II S-H* fractures are most commonly diagnosed on X-ray (Fig. 5.21); the fracture involves the physis and continues up through a small section of the metaphysis. This fracture is triangle-like and the periosteal layer is torn on the opposite side of the metaphyseal injury, but it is still intact on the adjacent side: the so-called Thurston-Holland sign (Fig. 5.22). After immobilization, healing is usually quick and complications are uncommon [33, 38]. *Type III S-H* fractures run along the joint surface and persist deep into the epiphyseal plate; they are relatively uncommon and usually they involve the distal tibial or peroneal

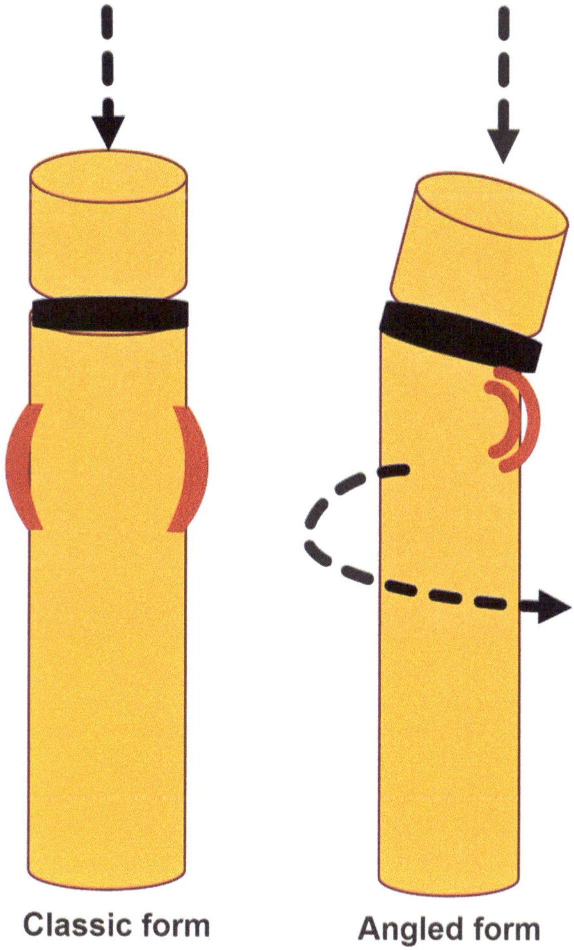

Fig. 5.16 A drawing representing the mechanism of injury in the buckle fractures. In the classic form, an axial loading (*dashed arrow*) results in a transverse, buckle fracture with an outward cortical bulging. In the angled form the same axial loading forces (*vertical dashed arrow*) are present, but other associated rotational forces (*angled dashed arrow*) result in a unilateral compression along the metaphysis and angulation of the cortex

bone (Fig. 5.23). A surgical approach is often required to ensure proper alignment of the fragments. However, the prospect of recovery is positive as long as the vascular supply to the bone remains intact [19, 33]. *Type IV S-H* fractures start above the growth plate, in the metaphysis, and cut all the way through the epiphysis (Fig. 5.24); these fractures are usually caused by axial loading or shear stress and comminution is common. Since these fractures damage the joint cartilage, the normal growth of the individual may be impaired and surgery is required in order to properly realign the joint surface [19]. *Type V* S-H fractures consist in a crushing of the physis; this is the hardest fracture type to diagnose and most difficult to heal. This injury is most likely to occur in the weight-bearing joints of the knee and ankle (Fig. 5.25). Crush injuries result in the disruption of the epiphyseal vascular system and in the death of the growth plate cartilage; this is why type V fractures always have an increased risk of premature fusion [22, 39, 40].

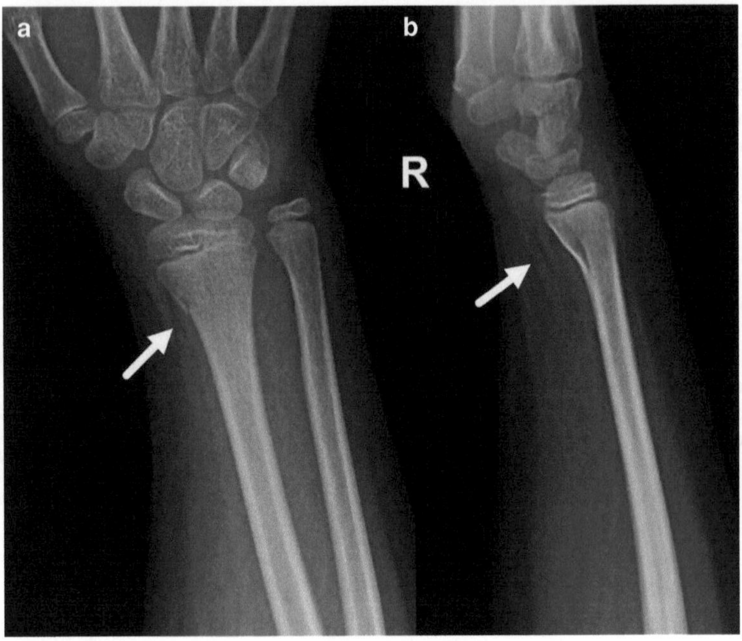

Fig. 5.17 Greenstick fracture. Female, 8 years old, slipped while walking on a wet board. The anterior (**a**) and the lateral (**b**) plain films reveal a greenstick fracture (*arrows*) of the right, distal, and radial metaphyses. A swelling of the adjacent soft tissues is also present

5.4 Birth Fractures

Fetal injuries are rare in both vaginal and cesarean deliveries and they usually do not have late consequences and are rarely associated with neurological trauma [11, 22]. The most common type involves the clavicle, but fracture of the long bones such as the humerus and femur, Monteggia fracture-dislocation, and rib fracture have been reported. In the clavicle most cases, the injury involves the middle third of the shaft, while when the distal third is fractured, it might be the result of a non-accidental trauma. The fracture may be incomplete or complete and closed or open, and usually the diagnosis is made through plain film or ultrasonography, the latter being the favorite in order to avoid X-ray exposure [35]. The risk factors for a birth fracture are maternal age, birth weight, prolonged labor, prematurity, macrosomia, malpresentation, shoulder dystocias, cephalopelvic disproportion, forceps-assisted delivery, and obstetric maneuvers in cesarean section (even if it is usually considered to be safer). When fetal injuries occur, it is important to exclude metabolic diseases such as osteogenesis imperfecta. Birth fracture usually heals very quickly and the fibrocartilage callus is complete in 7–12 days [6, 12, 16].

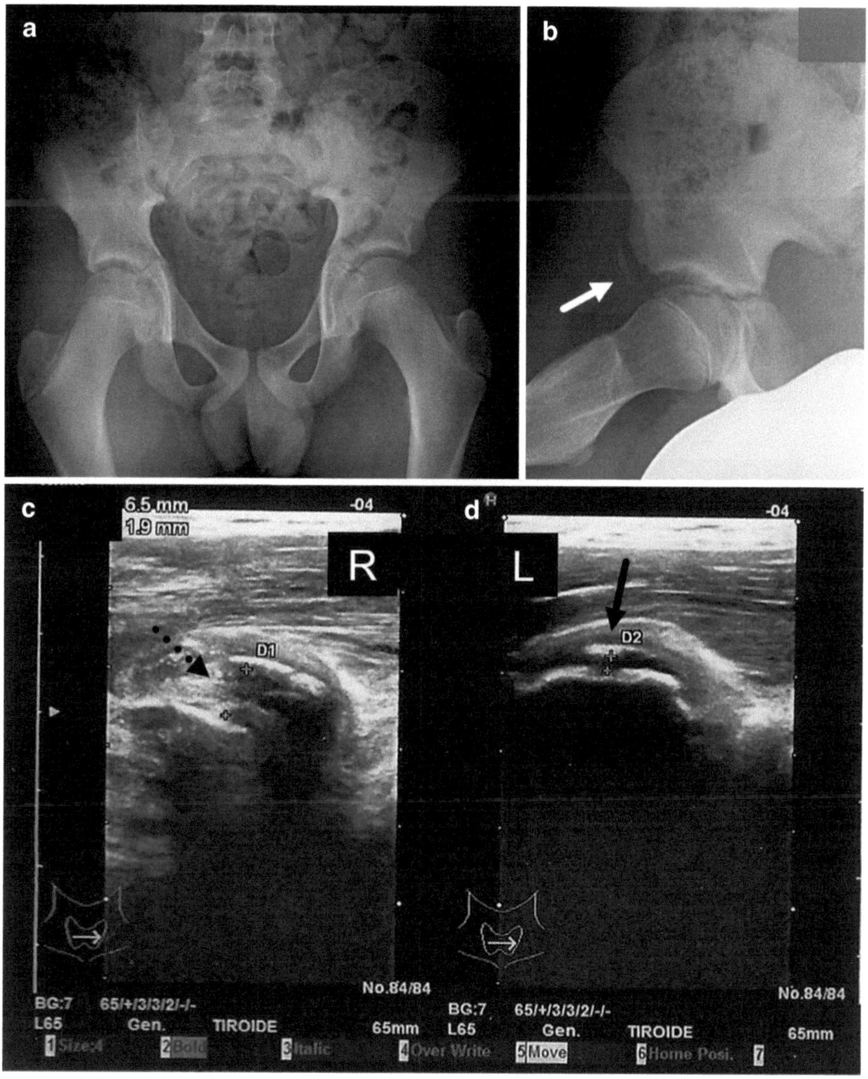

Fig. 5.18 Apophyseal injury of the right anterior-inferior iliac spine (AIIS) in a 12-year- old boy during a soccer game, after a wide kicking. The ultrasonographic examination (using a linear, 7.5 MHz probe), performed after the arrival of the young patient in the emergency department, shows an avulsion of the right AIIS (**c**, *dashed arrow*) and a normal AIIS on the other side (**d**, *arrow*). The AIIS is the insertion of rectus femoris muscle. In the following radiographic examination, the spine avulsion is well appreciable only in the oblique plain film (**b**, *arrow*) while the anterior plain film is near normal (**a**)

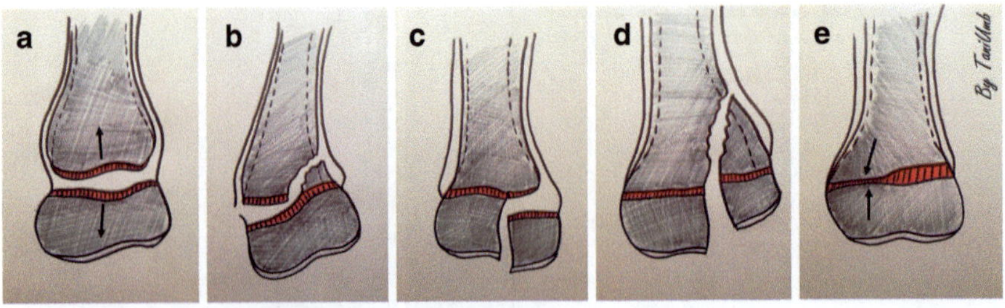

Fig. 5.19 A drawing representing the Salter-Harris (S-H) classification system of the physeal injuries. S-H type 1: complete separation of the entire physis (*arrow*) (**a**). S-H type 2 (**b**). S-H type 3 (**c**). S-H type 4 (**d**). S-H type 5: crushing of the physis (*arrow*) (**e**)

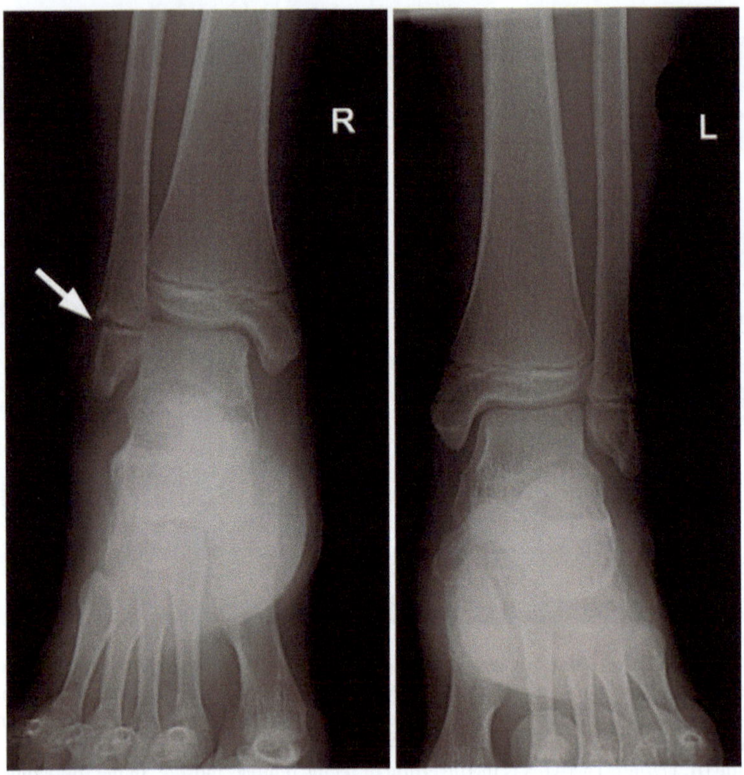

Fig. 5.20 Salter-Harris type 1 fracture. Female, 10 years old, after ankle sprain. The comparative radiographs of the tibiotarsal joint show a physeal injury with diastasis of the growth plate of the right peroneal malleolus (*arrow*)

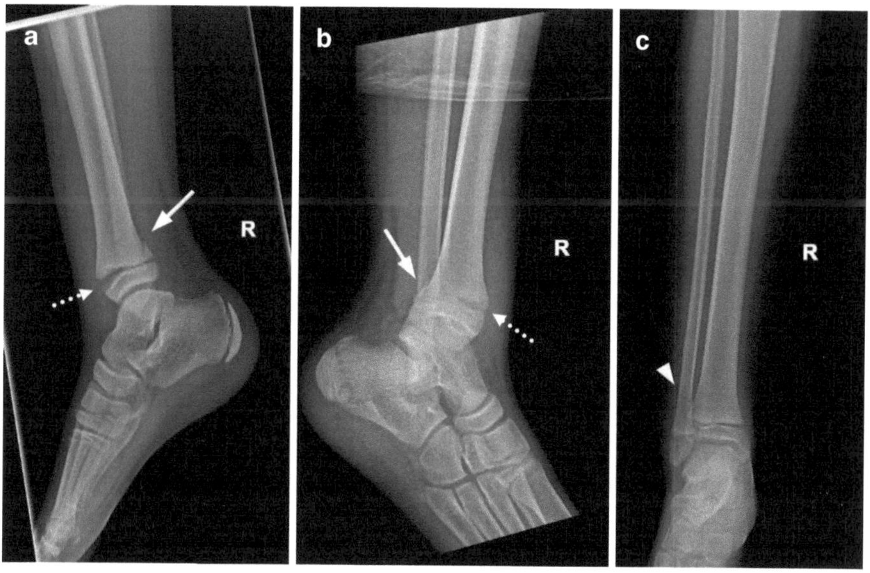

Fig. 5.21 Salter-Harris type 2 fracture. Female 9 years old. The lateral and oblique X-rays (respectively, in **a**, **b**) show an injury of the right distal tibial physis (*dashed arrow*) which continues up through a small section of the metaphysis (*arrow*). In the anterior plain film (**c**), only a right peroneal distal shaft fracture is clearly appreciable (*arrowhead*)

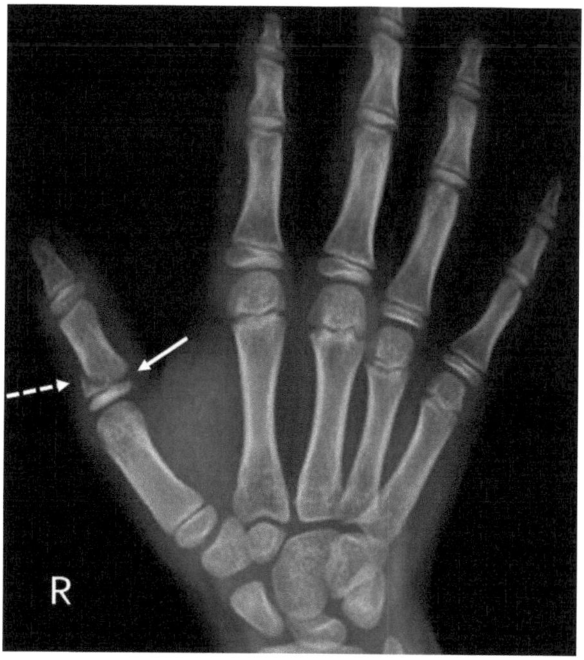

Fig. 5.22 Salter-Harris type 2 fracture. Male, 9 years old, injured while playing basketball. The anterior plain film shows a fracture of the proximal phalanx of the thumb with a physeal injury (*arrow*) and a metaphyseal fracture (*dashed arrow*)

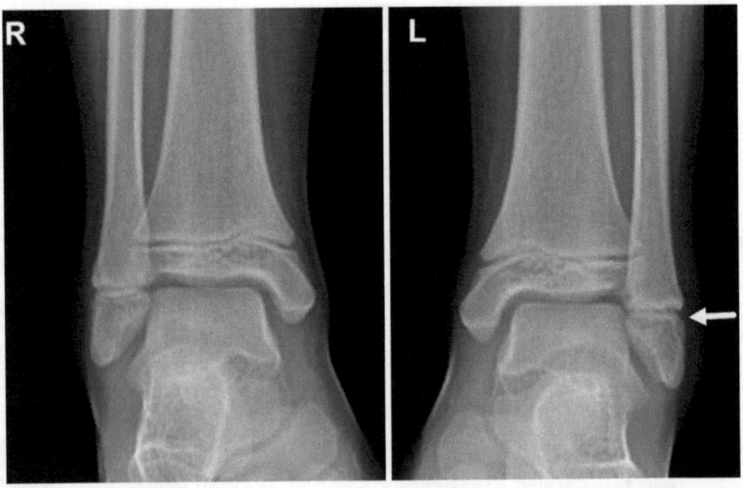

Fig. 5.23 Salter-Harris type 3 fracture. Female, 9 years old, pain after ankle sprain. The anterior comparative X-ray of ankles shows a fracture that runs along the joint surface into the epiphyseal plate of the left peroneal malleolus (*arrow*)

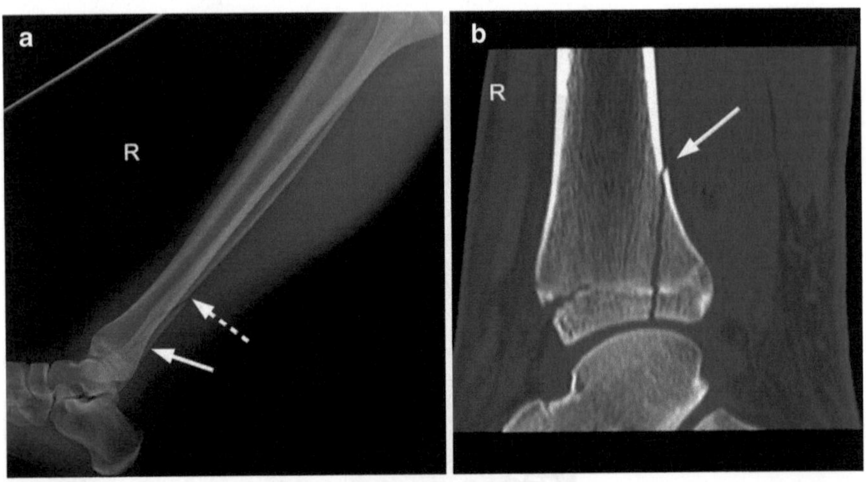

Fig. 5.24 Salter-Harris type 4 fracture. Male, 16 years old, injured during a soccer tackle. The lateral plain film (**a**) of the right ankle shows an oblique fracture of the peroneal shaft (*dashed arrow*) and an injury of the distal tibial metaphysis and epiphysis can be hardly perceived (*arrow*). Then a CT study was performed (**b**) and the Salter-Harris type 4 fracture (*arrow*) is better displayed

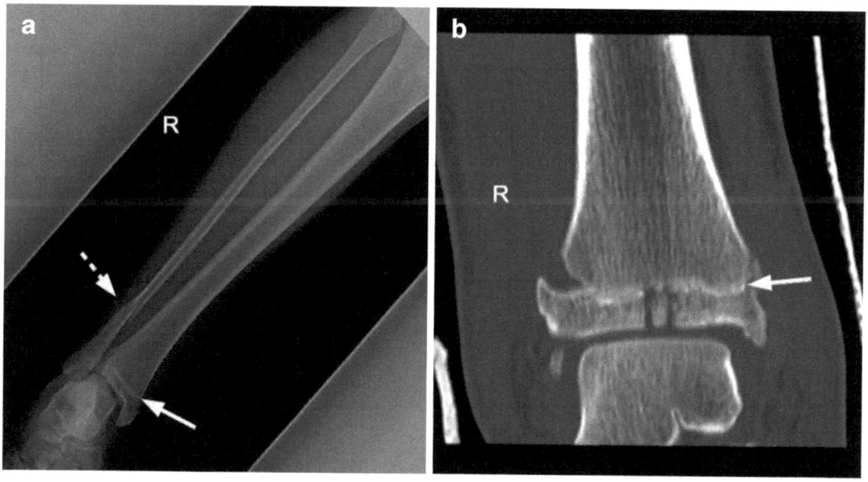

Fig. 5.25 Salter-Harris type 5 fracture. Female, 15 years old, ankle sprain while dancing. The anterior plain film (**a**) shows a fracture of the third distal of peroneal diaphysis (*dashed arrow*) and a Salter-Harris type 5 fracture (*arrow*) which is better appreciable in the CT scan executed subsequently (**b**)

5.5 Differences Between Pediatric and Adult Fracture Healing

The *fracture remodeling* is a process that occurs over several months following injury as a child's bone reshapes itself to an anatomic position. The amount of remaining bone growth provides the basis for remodeling. So the younger the child, the greater remodeling potential and the less important reduction accuracy is. The factors influencing the amount of remodeling are the age (younger children have greater remodeling potential), the location (fractures adjacent to the physis are associated with a greater amount of remodeling), the degree of deformity, and the plane of deformity with respect to the adjacent joint (remodeling occurs more readily in the plane of a joint than with deformity not in the plane of the joint) [12, 16, 22]. *Overgrowth* is a growth acceleration caused by physeal stimulation from the hyperemia associated with fracture healing and it is prominent in long bones (e.g., femur and humerus). It is usually present for 6 months to 1 year following injury and it does not present a continued progressive evolution unless complicated by a rare arteriovenous malformation. If the child is older than 10 years, the overgrowth is less of a problem and anatomic alignment is recommended [7, 9, 40]. *Progressive deformity* with growth is the complication of a physeal injury and the most common cause is a complete or partial closure of growth plates. Deformities can include angular deformity, shortening of bone, or both. Its magnitude depends upon the physis involved and the amount of growth remaining. The rapid healing of pediatric fractures (faster than adult ones) is due to children's growth potential and a thicker, more active periosteum, which contributes to the largest part of new bone formation around a fracture. As children reach their growth potential, in adolescence and early adulthood, the rate of healing slows to that of an adult. The downside of the rapid healing is a refracture [9, 15, 22, 25].

5.6 Clinical Evaluation

The initial approach to pediatric fractures includes a thorough history and physical exam. The clinicians must keep in mind that a young child may not be able to describe bone pain or the circumstances of injury [2, 3, 6]. As a consequence the toddlers and nonverbal children may simply present with the refusal to weight bear or move the injured area, with irritability, or with a new deformity observed by the caregivers. The history of a child presenting with a suspected fracture includes: (1) the characterization of the pain and presenting symptom; (2) location (is it the pain localized to a particular region or does it involve a larger area?); (3) intensity (use a pain scale from one to ten); (4) quality, onset, duration, and progress of pain (is it static, increasing, or decreasing? Is it the pain radiating? Is there any aggravating or "alleviating factors?); and (5) research of indicators of compromised neurovascular status (e.g., change in or loss of sensation, cold, pale, paralyzed limb). Other important considerations are the mechanism of injury; the possibility of non-accidental injury or child abuse, particularly in a child with limited physical mobility, with an injury out of proportion to the mechanism, with multiple injuries, or with a suspicious mechanism of injury (e.g., a 2-month-old baby who developmentally cannot roll, but who "rolled off the changing table"); and the rare possibility of an underlying bone abnormality (family history of fractures, bone or collagen disorders, prior fractures, mechanism out of proportion to injury). Physical examination should always include the assessment of the joint in question and, whenever non-accidental injury may be a possibility, a screening exam of the entire skeleton, fundoscopy, as well as an abdominal and cutaneous appraisal for signs of trauma [12, 17]. A joint above and below the symptomatic one should always be evaluated. The important features to include in the examination of all fractures are inspection; patient movement; discrepancy in limb length; palpation; assessment of local temperature, warmth, and tenderness; existence of swelling or mass; tightness, spasticity, and contracture; bone or joint deformity; evaluation of anatomic axis of the limb; active and passive range of motion of the joint; neurovascular condition of the injured area (inspection of the color of the limb; palpation for pulses and eliciting appropriate sensation to touch; temperature); and, if possible, estimation of strength in neighboring muscle groups. Finally, plain radiographs are the first step in evaluating most musculoskeletal disorders. When indicated, advanced imaging may include nuclear bone sans, ultrasonography, CT, MRI, and PET scans [5, 12, 24, 32, 35].

References

1. Huurman WH, Ginsburg GM (1997) Musculoskeletal injury in children. Pediat Rev 18(12):429–441
2. Slongo TF (2014) The pediatric patient. In: Smith WR, Stahel PF (ed) The management of the musculoskeletal injuries in the trauma patients. Springer, Germany, pp 29–84
3. Weber BG, Brunner C (1980) Treatment of fractures in children and adolescents. Springer, New York
4. Swischuk LE (2007) The limping infant: imaging and clinical evaluation of trauma. Emerg Radiol 14:219–226
5. Jenny C (2006) Evaluating infants and young children with multiple fractures. Pediatr Rev 118(3):1299–1303
6. Wright GJ, Young NL (2009) Outcome assessment in children with fractures. In: Green NE, Swiontkowski MF (eds) Skeletal trauma in children, 4th edn. Saunders/Elsevier, Philadelphia, pp 143–164
7. Peterson HA (2007) Epiphyseal Growyh plate fractures. Springer, Berlin
8. Hefti F, Brunner R, Freuler F, Hasler C, Jundt G (2007) Pediatric orthopedics in practice. Springer, Berlin
9. Johnstone EW, Foster BK (2001) The biological aspect of children's fractures. In: Rockwood CA, Wilkins KE, Beaty JH (eds) Rockwood and Wilkins' fractures in children, 5th edn. Lippincott Williams & Wilkins, Philadelphia, pp 22–35
10. Miller E, Davila J, Rotaru C, Koujok K (2012) Pediatric skeletal trauma. In: Donovan A, Schweitzer M (eds) Imaging musculoskeletal trauma: interpretation and reporting. Wiley-Blackwell, Chichester, pp 31–59
11. Martino F, Defilippi C, Caudana R (2011) Major traumatic bone and joint injuries: overview – imaging of pediatric bone and joint trauma. Springer, Berlin
12. Haller JO, Slovis TL, Joshi A (2005) Pediatric radiology, 3rd edn. Springer, Berlin/New York
13. Mabrey JD, Fitch RD (1989) Plastic deformation in pediatric fractures: mechanism and treatment. J Pediatr Orthop 9:310–314
14. Williams H (2007) Normal anatomical variants and other mimics of skeletal trauma. In: Bache E, Johnson KJ (eds) Imaging in pediatric skeletal trauma. Springer, Berlin/London, pp 91–117
15. Currey JD, Butler G (1975) The mechanical properties of bone tissue in children. J Bone Joint Surg Am 57:810–814
16. Bache E, Johnson KJ (2007) Basic science of pediatric fractures. In: Bache E, Johnson KJ (eds) Imaging in pediatric skeletal trauma. Springer, Berlin/London, pp 119–131
17. Jadhav SP, Swischuk LE (2014) Emergency musculoskeletal imaging in children. Springer, New York
18. Blount WP (1968) Fractures in children. Lippincott Williams & Wilkins, Baltimore
19. Salter RB (1999) Textbook of disorders and injuries of the musculoskeletal system. Lippincott Williams & Wilkins, Baltimore
20. Rogers LE, Malave S Jr, White H, Tachdjian MO (1978) Plastic bowing, torus and greenstick supracondylar fractures of the humerus: radiographic cues to obscure fractures of the elbow in children. Radiology 128:145–150
21. Goswami GK (2002) The fat pad sign. Radiology 222:419–420
22. Frick SL, Jones ET (2009) Skeletal growth, development and healing as related to pediatric trauma. In: Green NE, Swiontkowski MF (eds) Skeletal trauma in children, 4th edn. Saunders/Elsevier, Philadelphia, pp 1–26
23. Dolan M, Waters PM (2009) Fractures and dislocations of the forearm, wrist and hand. In: Green NE, Swiontkowski MF (eds) Skeletal trauma in children, 4th edn. Saunders/Elsevier, Philadelphia, pp 159–211
24. Laor T, Jaramillo D, Oestreich AE (1998) Musculoskeletal system. In: Kirks DR (ed) Practical pediatric imaging, 3rd edn. Lippincott- Raven, Philadelphia, pp 427–433

25. Calmar A, Vinci RJ (2002) The anatomy and physiology of bone fracture and healing. Clin Pediatr Emerg Med 3(2):86–93
26. Judet J, Judet R, Lefranc J (1962) Fracture du col radial chez l'enfant. Ann Chir 16:1377–1385
27. Stiefel D, Meuli M, Altermatt S (2001) Fractures of the neck of the radius in children. J Bone Joint Surg 83-B:536–541
28. Siddharth PJ, Swischuk LE (2008) Commonly missed subtle skeletal injuries in children: a pictorial review. Emerg Radiol 15:391–398
29. Tschoepe EJ, John SD, Swischuk LE (1998) Tibial fractures in infants and children: emphasis on subtle injuries. Emerg Radiol 5(4):245–252
30. Swischuk LE, Hernadez JA (2004) Frequently missed fractures in children (value of comparative views). Emerg Radiol 11:22–28
31. Hernandez JA, Swischuk LE, Yngve DA, Carmichael KD (2003) The angled buckle fracture in pediatrics: a frequently missed fracture. Emerg Radiol 10:71–75
32. Kerssemakers SP, Fotiadou AN, De Jonge MC et al (2009) Sport injuries in the paediatric and adolescent patient: a growing problem. Pediatr Radiol 39(5):471–484
33. Papadonikolakis A, Li Z, Smith PB et al (2006) Fractures of the phalanges and interphalangeal joints in children in pediatric fractures dislocations and sequelae. Hand Clin 22:133–136
34. Kumar R, Swischuk LE, Madewell GE (1986) Benign cortical defect: site for an avulsion fracture. Skeletal Radiol 15:553–555
35. O'Connor PJ, Groves C (2005) Trauma and sports related injuries. In: Wilson D (ed) Paediatric musculoskeletal disease with an emphasis on ultrasound. Springer, Berlin, pp 19–37
36. Jadhav SP, Swischuk LE (2008) Commonly subtle missed skeletal injuries in children: a pictorial review. Emerg Radiol 15:391–398
37. Burnei G, Gavrilliu S, Georgescu I et al (2010) The therapeutic attitude in distal radial Salter and Harris type I and II fractures in children. J Med Life 3(1):70–75
38. Izadpanah A, Karunanayake M, Izadpanah A et al (2012) Salter-Harris type 2 fracture of the proximal phalanx of the thumb with a rotational deformity: a case report and review. Pediatr Emerg Care 28(3):288–289
39. Wilkins KE, Aroojis AJ (2001) The present status of children's fractures. In: Rockwood CA, Wilkins KE, Beaty JH (eds) Rockwood and Wilkins' fractures in children, 5th edn. Lippincott Williams & Wilkins, Philadelphia, pp 8–19
40. Laer LV (2004) Pediatric fractures and dislocations. Thieme, Stuttgart/New York

6 Ultrasound and Magnetic Resonance Imaging of Pediatric Musculoskeletal Injuries

Michele Galluzzo, Claudia Piccolo, Grazia Loretta Buquicchio, Riccardo Palliola, and Margherita Trinci

6.1 Introduction

Medical and diagnostic evaluation of musculoskeletal trauma, together with epidemiologic data, is a complex issue for several aspects.

Firstly, it is because of the anatomy and physiological changes of the musculoskeletal system during physical and psycho-attitudinal growth.

Around 10–15 % of the overall pediatric traumas are represented by musculoskeletal injuries.

Around 40 % of the musculoskeletal traumas in the young population are sports-related, involving mostly male patients (2:1).

During the child's growth, the characteristics of the musculoskeletal apparatus are unique, so it is necessary and important to know the anatomy and physiological changes during the growth in order to better understand and evaluate injuries and to perform the most adequate and correct management.

It is known that an erroneous diagnosis and further mishandling of orthopedic pediatric injuries may cause future disabilities in the patient.

X-ray imaging represents the first technique of choice for the study of the bone component, even though it is not fully satisfying with respect to soft tissue injuries.

Ultrasound (US) and magnetic resonance imaging (MRI) are the main imaging modalities in studying and approaching issues concerning tendons, ligaments, muscles, and osteochondral cartilage.

M. Galluzzo (✉) • C. Piccolo • G.L. Buquicchio • R. Palliola • M. Trinci
Cardiovascular and Emergency Radiology Department, S. Camillo Hospital, C.ne Gianicolense, 87, Rome, 00152, Italy
e-mail: mgalluzzo@scamilloforlanini.rm.it; c.piccolo@unicampus.it; graziabuquicchio@gmail.com; palliola@libero.it; margherita.trinci@libero.it

V. Miele, M. Trinci (eds.), *Imaging Trauma and Polytrauma in Pediatric Patients*, DOI 10.1007/978-3-319-08524-1_6

Every year, a quarter of the child population goes to the emergency department for an orthopedic trauma.

During early childhood, most traumas are caused by falls (1/3) and car accidents (1/5), especially for young children involved in pedestrian and bike-riding accidents, and later on, teenagers are involved in trauma during sports activities (1/10), at an amateur or competitive level.

The increasing incidence of sports trauma is due to the increase of the number of young people doing sports activity and of the number of sport/fitness centers.

Furthermore, sports activity is often suggested by pediatrics in helping the child's physical and psycho-attitudinal growth, in strengthening self-confidence, and for possibilities of creating new relationships and friends. This is often supported by the family that considers the success in sports as an improvement in their child's future social life.

The basic principle is that a child is not "a small adult" and traumatic injury and radiological appearance can be different in childhood from that in other ages.

In all young athletes, but mainly in those that play sports at a competitive level, an early diagnosis of the injury allows to determine the recovery period and allows the patient to start playing sports again in the best possible safety conditions.

This is why diagnostic imaging plays a very important role in this given scenario, thanks to the use of different types of techniques, allowing to confirm clinical data and evaluate the follow-up of the lesion.

Another important topic is that the musculoskeletal system can be affected, in both acute and chronic injury, by different and simultaneous lesions, such as muscle trauma contusions (of different degrees), tendon and/or ligament injuries, fracture or joint dislocation, frequently in combination between them.

Several imaging modalities are used in sports medicine.

Ultrasound has many positive aspects: basically easy to use, inexpensive, widely used, and totally safe.

The radiologist who carries out the musculoskeletal ultrasound is highly supported by an "interactive" method with the patient, which allows to depict and locate the involved area in real time and carry out comparative views and dynamic maneuvers eventually by using power Doppler, useful for the muscular injury follow-up.

This method has a high-level sensibility in muscular injuries (distraction, contusion), both tendinous and ligamentous (75 % sensibility and 90 % specificity), and in evaluating superficial hematoma.

The main limit of ultrasound is to be strongly dependent by the physician so it is necessary for radiologists, handling musculoskeletal injuries, to have confidence with it, and be supported by an important background experience and knowledge skill in clinical cases concerning pediatric pathologies.

Thanks to its high spatial and contrast resolution, MR imaging is a method that allows to carry out a detailed and complete study on tendinous, cartilaginous, and osteochondral components, all issues in which an injury is suspected and where first-level exams are inconclusive.

Furthermore, MRI being without radiation exposure, it is particularly recommended in the "management" of pediatric patients especially in young athletes that must undergo follow-ups after traumatic injury in the monitoring of complete "restitutio ad integrum."

6.2 Upper Limb

6.2.1 Clavicle Fractures

Clavicle fracture is the most common fracture of the child owing to its superficial anatomical position.

It may occur during natural childbirth in high-weight children or during a difficult delivery, generally at the level of the middle-distal third, due to the pressure of the shoulder against the symphysis pubis in the ejection phase.

An anteroposterior radiograph can easily be achieved for the diagnosis, but also ultrasonography can be useful to highlight the discontinuity of the bone heads in those cases of incomplete lesions and in the follow-ups.

Ultrasound may be usefull.

In older children, they are due to trauma from a fall with the arm in extension or to a side impact.

The most common site is the middle third, the less flexible point (75–80 %), then the lateral third (15–20 %), and the medial bone (5 %) [1].

Clinically, pain with any shoulder movement and upon holding the arm across the chest and tenderness over the fracture can be observed.

In the third side fractures, the latter one is displaced downward owing to the weight of the arm and to the action of the pectoralis major and latissimus dorsi muscles, while in third-medium fractures, the bone fragment is displaced upward by the action of the sternocleidomastoid muscle.

Complications are rare but they must be recognized as the damage of the neurovascular bundle or pleuropulmonary lesions may occur.

In case of more complex injuries or when it is associated with a sternoclavicular joint dislocation, CT is indicated, especially CT angiography, to rule out potential vascular injury.

Sternoclavicular joint dislocation is anterosuperior in 90 % and posterior in the remaining 10 %; it is difficult to diagnose on plain radiographs and it can be associated with other complications.

Nonunion is common in clavicle fractures that occur distal to the attachment of the coracoclavicular ligament.

Stress or "academic" clavicular fractures may be seen in students who carry heavy loads of books on their shoulders.

Acromioclavicular joint dislocation represents 12 % of all shoulder injuries, and it is more common than clavicular ones (98 %) and has been subdivided into six types of growing instability.

US is very useful and more sensitive than x-ray, especially in low-grade lesions.

6.2.2 Shoulder: Acute Injuries

Children acute shoulder fractures commonly involve the proximal humeral and scapular aspect. Most of them are clearly diagnosed by x-ray. However, avulsion fractures in the coracoid and glenoid growth center are more difficult to detect by radiographs, and in these cases, US or MRI might be necessary for the diagnosis [2] (Fig. 6.1).

The addition of several imaging modalities can be useful also for the diagnosis of preexisting pathologies (Fig. 6.2).

Traumatic glenohumeral dislocations usually occur in collision sports, such as football and hockey. It is a disorder of the growing-up age, and about 40 % of these occur in patients under the age of 22, although it is uncommon in younger children, with only 1.6 % seen in patients under the age of 10 years [3, 4].

Recurrent dislocation and glenohumeral instability are common after a first-time dislocation and have the highest incidence in patients with open physis.

Most glenohumeral dislocations are anterior with the humerus abducted and externally rotated at the time of the impact with anteroinferior aspect of the humeral head.

The labro-ligamentous complex can be avulsed from the glenoid (classic Bankart lesion) with or without disruption (distacco) of the adjacent scapular periosteum or with bony glenoid fracture (bony Bankart).

The impact of the posterolateral aspect of the humeral head may create a visible depression in the humeral head (Hill-Sachs defect), seen in 38–90 % of patients [5].

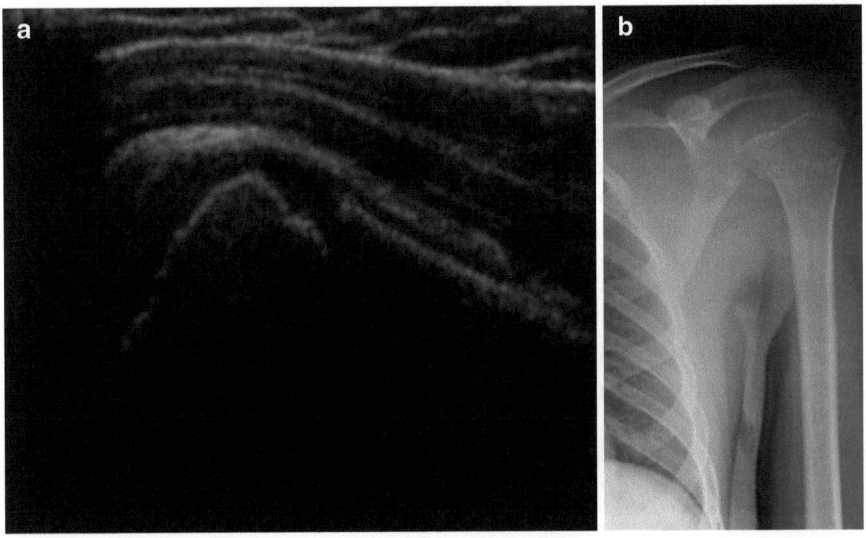

Fig. 6.1 (**a**) Longitudinal US view of the left shoulder of an 8-year-old girl performed for acute humeral pain shows an irregularity of the cortical aspect of the proximal humerus. (**b**) Anteroposterior view shows a fracture of the proximal physis, which accounts for the longitudinal growth of the humerus

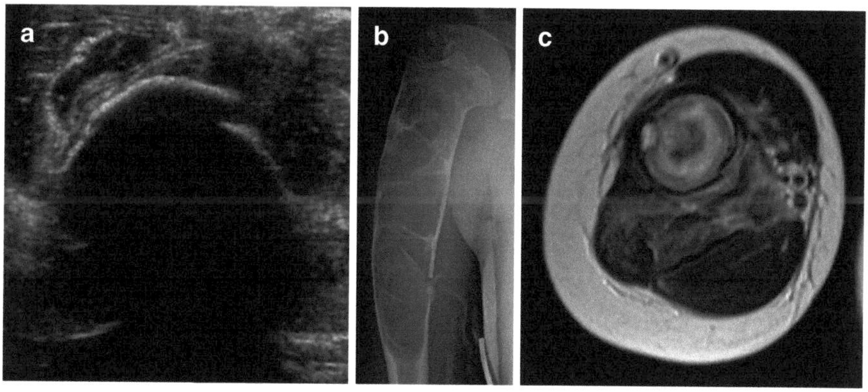

Fig. 6.2 A young female patient with a history of a known juvenile bone cyst presenting with acute pain after a fall. (**a**) US shows irregularity of the cortical zone. (**b**) Anteroposterior view of the right shoulder confirmed the cyst rupture with cortical interruption. (**c**) Axial T2-weighted image highlights the presence of a double-density fluid-level lesion within the bone, associated with an inhomogeneous intensity of adjacent soft tissue, appearing edematous and inflamed

Hill-Sachs defect is associated with a higher incidence of recurrence (82 % vs 50 %) [3, 6, 7].

In patients with recurrent instability, a more detailed imaging is mandatory.

A great deal of soft tissue capsulolabral injuries associated with acute or chronic recurrent dislocations or instability and diagnosis is best provided by MRI.

Many authors agree that MR arthrography is the most accurate technique, with the greatest efficacy in the younger, athletic population [8, 9] and an overall sensitivity of 91 % for the detection of labral pathology.

HAGL lesion (humeral avulsion of the glenohumeral ligament) is very important to recognize on MRI; the anterior band of the inferior glenohumeral ligament is torn from its humeral neck attachment and can be seen on MRI as a "J" sign.

About two-thirds of HAGL lesions are associated with other shoulder pathologies, such as labral tears, rotator cuff tears, and Hill-Sachs alterations [10, 11].

Failure to recognize these types of lesions leads to recurrent instability; MR diagnosis is important in surgical planning [11].

Ultrasound has a poor indication in cases of instability; therefore, in these cases, it can be useful in the assessment of fluid collection or indirect signs of instability at the level of the long head of the biceps, the glenohumeral ligament, or the acromioclavicular joint.

Posterior dislocation is less common, and it usually occurs with an axial loading of an adducted internally rotated arm, violent muscle contraction, or posterior glenoid deficiency, as occurs in brachial plexus palsy [12].

MRI is usually performed in order to evaluate the presence of a posterior labral tear, a capsular rent, a "reverse" Hill-Sachs, or an abnormal glenoid version [13, 14].

Superior labral anterior to posterior (SLAP) tears occurring in children are due to microtrauma associated with overhead throwing or are traumatic. In throwers, they are caused by the increased external rotation during the cocking phase, producing enormous torsional stresses at the biceps anchor and the superior labrum causing the detachment of the labrum medially, over the corner of the glenoid.

Another cause of SLAP tears in throwers is the internal impingement; it occurs when the arm is abducted and externally rotated, as we have in the cocking phase, leading to repetitive contact between the humeral and the posterosuperior aspect of the glenoid.

In addition may be those traumas producing traction or compression on the biceps anchor, such as a fall onto an outstretched arm [15, 16].

MRI is mandatory in SLAP tears when surgery is planned; typical MR findings consist of rotator cuff tears, anterior and posterior labral tears, paralabral cysts, and chondral injuries.

MRI can recognize the normal variants of the anterior labrum: the superior sublabral recess, the sublabral foramen, and the Buford complex [17].

MRI can recognize the presence of a paralabral or spinoglenoid notch cyst, associated with persistent symptoms and failure of nonoperative treatment in children with SLAP tears, or compression of the suprascapular nerve and denervation of the infraspinatus [18].

6.2.3 Shoulder: Chronic Repetitive Trauma

Repetitive stress is the leading cause of shoulder injuries in younger athletes. Most of them are observed during the mid to the late teen years, due to the increase of stress forces applied to muscular structures in this age group. These particular conditions have been often observed in baseball players but also in football, swimming, tennis, and all those sports requiring an overhead activity [19].

Little leaguer's shoulder is a descriptive term used to refer to a stress-related injury of the proximal humeral physis, characterized by the epiphysiolysis of the proximal humeral growth plate.

It usually occurs in 11- to 16-year-olds, presenting with dominant arm shoulder pain aggravated by throwing and tenderness to palpation.

This condition affects those athletes who frequently repeat the action of overhead throwing, such as baseball players, track-and-field athletes, only later volleyball players, tennis players, and swimmers. It is a benign and self-limited condition responding well to conservative treatment [20].

It is characterized by the widening and irregularity of the proximal humeral physis, easily detectable both on x-ray and MRI, which can also highlight the logistic aspect as an area of high signal intensity on T2-weighted images [21].

Rotator cuff injuries are rare in children because the rotator cuff in young patients is more elastic and stronger, without the degenerative changes observed in the elderly population.

They usually occur as tendonitis or strain in response to repetitive microtrauma caused by overhead arm motion.

In younger athletes, rotator cuff injuries are often associated with joint instability [5, 22].

Primary impingement can occur as a result of a tight coracoacromial arch or simple overuse.

With repetitive stress, the muscle becomes weaker and rotator cuff impingement can result from a multidirectional instability.

These injuries are the major indicators for an ultrasound examination.

They can be classified as complete, incomplete, or partial (sensitivity: 91 %) [9].

Complete lesions extend over the whole thickness from the articular side to the bursal one, presenting hypo-anechoic focal areas with evidence of joint effusion within the coracoid and axillary recesses or in the anatomical locations of tendons. In complete rupture, the tendon is no longer recognizable and tucked beneath the coracoacromial arch.

Other described signs are the double cortex sign, the sagging peribursal fat sign, compressibility, and muscle atrophy.

A *partial lesion* is characterized by a hypo-anechoic area with poorly defined margins affecting only the articular or bursal portion of the tendon.

However, there is a spectrum of non-rotator cuff abnormalities that are amenable to US examination, including the instability of the biceps tendon, glenohumeral joint, and acromioclavicular joint; arthropathies and bursitis (inflammatory diseases, degenerative and infiltrative disorders, infections); nerve entrapment syndromes; and space-occupying lesions.

MRI is the modality of choice for the evaluation of rotator cuff tears.

When a tendinopathy occurs, it is easy to see an intermediate signal intensity on T2-weighted images within the tendon.

A full-thickness tear appears as a hyperintensity on T2-weighted images extending completely through the tendon. A complete tear disrupts the tendon completely, with musculotendinous retraction and a possible upward subluxation of the humeral head.

A partial-thickness tear may present both on the articular and bursal surface and appears as a hyperintensity on T2-weighted images extending through the tendon thickness, superiorly or inferiorly [23, 24].

A rim-rent tear is a partial articular tear of the insertional fibers of the rotator cuff at the greater tuberosity; it is considered as a form of partial rotator cuff tear, and it may involve both the supraspinatus and infraspinatus insertion. If left untreated, it may progress to a full-thickness tear [25].

Subscapularis tendon tears are less common and are frequently associated with biceps tendon abnormalities.

Internal impingement is characterized by the entrapment of the undersurface of the posterior supraspinatus tendon or anterior infraspinatus tendon between the humeral head and posterior glenoid. Undersurface tears of one or both tendons with cystic changes in the posterior humeral head and posterosuperior labral pathology are diagnostic for internal impingement [26].

In conclusion, once adequate radiographs have been obtained to exclude apparent bone disorders, high-resolution US should be the first-line imaging modality in the assessment of non-rotator cuff disorders, assuming the study is performed with high-end equipment by an experienced examiner. More costly and invasive modalities such as MR imaging and MR arthrography should be reserved for bone marrow evaluation and preoperative assessment.

6.2.4 Elbow: Acute Injuries

Pediatric elbow joint trauma is challenging and particularly complex mainly because of the complex anatomy and the presence of several growth plates appearing in different phases of the growing process.

In children, elbow trauma may lead to bony, cartilaginous, or soft tissue injury.

In most of cases, basic radiographs compared with the injured elbow can allow a complete evaluation of injuries, such as joint effusions or fractures, identifying injuries that require surgical intervention, obviating the need for multiplanar imaging.

A careful assessment of soft tissues can provide information about the presence of a possible fracture, because it is frequently associated with the presence of joint effusion.

In the L-L radiogram, when effusion is present, the "fat-pad sign," reported in 1954, will appear both anteriorly and posteriorly to the third distal aspect of the humerus.

When an anterior conspicuous dislocation of the fat pad is observed, it will result in the classic "sign of the sail," which is very important because about 90 % of young patients with these radiographic features have a fracture of the elbow. The posterior humeral fat pad is not visible on a normal elbow and becomes visible in the presence of joint effusion.

However, x-ray does not show bone bruising or cartilaginous or soft tissue injury and may underestimate physeal injury, as demonstrated by Beltran and Rosenberg [27] who reported, in a study comprising of eight patients with elbow fractures, that two children had unsuspected transphyseal fracture extension through the unossified epiphyseal cartilage shown by MR imaging.

Carey et al. [28] reported that in 14 suspected physeal injuries, MRI changed the radiographic diagnosis in 50 % of the cases by showing either radiographically occult fractures or unsuspected transphyseal extension. MR findings resulted in a change of treatment in 36 % of the cases.

MRI can improve the understanding of complex trauma; confirm the presence of an occult fracture suggested just by a joint effusion on x-ray; show the condition of the surrounding musculotendinous structures, such as the insertion of biceps muscle upon the radial tuberosity; and evaluate the ulnar nerve, because of its path posteriorly around the medial epicondyle.

In fact, as demonstrated by Major and Crawford, MRI highlighted marrow edema and missed fractures in 13 patients whose initial posttraumatic elbow showed just a joint effusion without fracture [29].

In children of less than 2 years, before the mineralization of secondary growth plates, bony landmarks are not present, limiting the accuracy of x-rays. On the contrary, MRI may easily visualize the unossified growth plate and the cartilage, providing a good contrast between joint fluid, cartilage, and ossified bone [30].

The joint is well assessed by ultrasound which allows the evaluation of tendons, ligaments, muscles, and neurovascular components.

It also allows the assessment of any intra-articular body and the search for any incomplete fracturative lesion where painful swelling is visible.

Pediatric elbow injuries are commonly classified as lateral compression, medial tension overload, and extension overload depending on the mechanism of injury.

They typically occur during the acceleration phase of the throwing cycle when enormous forces are applied on the elbow joint.

In fact, during this phase, compressive forces are applied laterally, across the radiocapitellar joint; tensile forces are exerted medially across the ulnar collateral ligament and flexor/pronator muscle group; posterior tensile forces are applied as the triceps muscle contracts; and impaction forces are exerted as the olecranon extends into the olecranon fossa [31].

Some authors described that about 17–20 % of baseball pitchers between 9 and 15 years of age experience elbow pain during their careers. The incidence of elbow injuries is directly correlated with pitching frequency and is higher for pitchers who throw with poor technique [32–34].

Acute elbow injuries in the pediatric age are not only a characteristic of sports activities; they often occur because of a fall onto an outstretched hand, seen within or outside the sports field.

Medial epicondylar avulsion fracture: It is common (12 % overall) and sometimes associated with the alteration of normal articular relations; they are classified into two types by Woods.

It often occurs among baseball pitchers (7–15 years old) as the medial epicondyle begins to fuse. It is the result of a violent valgus force exerted on the elbow during overhead throwing with a contemporary contraction of the flexor/pronator muscle group.

Radiography is often diagnostic, although US and MRI might be useful when we have an avulsed fracture fragment difficult to see on x-rays [35].

Ulnar collateral ligament (UCL) lesion: In an older adolescent with a fused epicondyle, the UCL may be torn, partially (involving the deep intracapsular layer of the anterior bundle) or completely (more common, involving the midsubstance of the anterior bundle) [36].

It is an uncommon injury and US and MRI can easily depict this kind of lesion.

On T2-weighted MRI sequences, a disruption of the ligament and wave aspect of the fibers and increased intensity can be noticed.

However, the radiologist must be careful about the interpretation of the high signal intensity at the origin of the ligament, because a mild increase of T2 signal intensity at the origin is normal also in the immature skeleton.

Partial tears occur at the ulnar insertion, and in this case, MRI shows the "T" sign, which is the high signal intensity at the distal site of the ligament.

Tendon lesions: They most commonly occur at the distal side of the biceps and at the insertion site of the triceps.

Biceps lesions typically occur during the teenage phase, and they are commonly due to a lift effort; they are well depicted by both US and MRI.

US evaluation can be challenging because of its complex anatomy.

It is important to evaluate also the contralateral elbow and to perform the dynamic tests.

The distal biceps tendon has no tendon sheath that lies in the anterior compartment of the elbow, superficial to the brachialis muscle. Its tendon passes through the antecubital fossa to insert on the radial tuberosity.

Ultrasound examination shows thickening of the tendon fibers, muscle retraction, and the presence of blood infarction.

Searching for the triceps tendon injuries, the comparative radiological evaluation of the elbow in L-L projection is critical; in addition, US is very useful for the diagnosis of complete and partial tears, providing an alternative to MR imaging [37, 38].

6.2.5 Elbow: Chronic Repetitive Trauma

During school age, the shoulder, elbow, and wrist can be susceptible to many sports-related overuse injuries.

Little leaguer's elbow: It is a term used to describe those injuries which affect the medial, lateral, and posterior compartments of the elbow of throwers and gymnasts, in which the "primum movens" is the repetitive valgus overload [39].

Classic little leaguer's elbow: During childhood and adolescence, the weakest site is the medial epicondyle physis, where chronic and repeated stress, aged by the common tendon of the flexor/pronator muscles and the ulnar collateral ligament, results in the irritation of the physeal cartilage. When it becomes chronic, it is easily detectable by the widening of the medial epicondyle physis, irregularity of the margins, and, eventually, sclerosis and fragmentation [40].

The most common radiographic manifestations are displacement and fragmentation of the medial epicondyle apophysis, although plain film can·be normal in up to 85 % of cases.

US and MRI are very useful, especially in those cases in which there is a high clinical suspicion but radiographs are normal.

Sonography has a great ability to medial epicondylar fragmentation.

The epicondyle shows a large area of marrow edema, the physis being widened and hyperintense on T2-weighted images; a thickening of common flexor tendon could also be shown.

Panner disease: It is an osteochondral lesion responsible for lateral elbow pain in children.

It is attributed to avascular necrosis of the capitellum and typically affects the dominant elbow of boys aged 5–12 years.

The onset age is younger than that of patients with osteochondritis dissecans (OCD), occurring during the period of active ossification of the capitellar epiphysis [41].

X-ray shows lucency adjacent to the capitellar articular surface with mild surrounding sclerosis. Days later, larger areas of capitellar radiolucency mixed with diffuse sclerotic changes are clearly visible.

MRI is much more sensitive than x-ray in the early detection of Panner disease; in fact, it can demonstrate diffuse capitellar marrow edema. Normalization of capitellar appearance usually occurs within 1–2 years.

Almost all patients affected by Panner disease recover well, with no treatment, and fully reconstitute the normal architecture of the capitellum.

Osteochondritis dissecans (OCD) of the capitellum: It typically occurs in older adolescents aged 11–15 years, when the capitellar epiphysis is almost completely ossified. It consists of a fragment of the capitellum separated or isolated from the surrounding bone. The cause is still unclear, but many authors suggest that it could be a combination of repetitive microtrauma across the radiocapitellar joint and the mild blood supply of the capitellum [41].

Baseball players and gymnasts are often affected by this condition, perhaps because of distraction forces across the medial elbow producing tension forces across the lateral joint.

OCD begins on the anterolateral aspect of the capitellum as a mild subchondral lucency, while Panner disease involves the entire ossification center.

Later on, there is an increasing process of lytic and sclerotic changes with the flattening and fragmentation of the capitellum. Advanced aspects of OCD are characterized by loose body formation, expansion of the radial head, and osteophyte formation.

Sonography is very sensitive to detect OCD capitellar fragmentation.

MRI spectrum of OCD is more severe than that of Panner disease, including abnormal marrow signal, cystic changes, cartilaginous defects, fragmentation, and intra-articular loose bodies.

Two patterns of OCD presentation have been described: one pattern shows a low-signal-intensity ring surrounded by an intermediate area on T1-weighted sequences; the inner portion of the ring is hyperintense on T2-weighted images. The second pattern is characterized by a segmental area of hypointensity on T1-weighted images, which is hyperintensity on T2-weighted ones.

The use of MRI arthrography with gadolinium improves the staging of osteochondral lesions; in fact, in unstable lesions, we observe some fluid or contrast agent encircling the fragment or a cystic lesion under the fragment on T2-weighted images.

MRI not only makes diagnosis and evaluates its extension and the possible presence of displaced fragments, but it can also assist with the evaluation of the stability of the lesion.

Stable lesions have a focus of low signal intensity on T1-weighted images and high signal intensity on T2-weighted images in a portion of the anterior capitellum.

MR instability criteria are a rim of high T2 signal intensity around the lesion, disruption of the subchondral bone plate, cartilage cracks around the lesion and cysts inside it, or displaced fragments [41].

The presence of intra-articular contrast material around the lesion suggests disruption of the articular surface, indicating the instability of the lesion.

Post-contrast MRI can also be used in order to evaluate patients affected by OCD. The use of i.v. gadolinium contrast may help assess the stability and viability of the lesion. In fact, enhancement of the lesion suggests that it is viable and with good blood supply. On the other hand, the presence of a ring of diffuse enhancement between the OCD lesion and adjacent subchondral bone might represent granulation tissue, indicating that the lesion is unstable.

The last component is the posterior elbow involvement. In fact, during throwing or tumbling, the triceps may impute strong traction on the olecranon, known as "extension overload," in which the first site affected is the olecranon physis. This condition is characterized by apophyseal widening, irregularity, and delayed closure.

6.2.6 Wrist and Hand: Acute Injuries

Plain film radiographs can provide a detailed evaluation of bone injuries, the degree of radial foreshortening, abnormalities or angulation of the distal radius, possible ulnar fracture or dislocation, and so on.

However, MRI allows additional evaluation of soft tissue supporting structures, especially the intercarpal ligaments and the triangular fibrocartilage (TFC).

TFC tears may occur not only as a long-term result of gymnast wrist or positive ulnar variance but also acutely. In younger athletes, traumatic injuries with respect to the degenerative ones are most common [42, 43].

TFC tears can be a partial-thickness defect or complete perforation through the entire thickness of the disk and can affect both the central (radial) side and the peripheral (ulnar) side. This distinction is important because it affects the treatment; in fact, tears of the ulnar side are repaired because of the rich vascular supply, while central tears are debrided [44].

Clinically, they manifest with ulnar-side wrist pain and a palpable click, associated also with swelling and loss of grip strength.

At MRI, a partial tear is characterized by an irregular or linear surface defect, whereas a complete tear or perforation shows a hyperintense linear abnormality on T2-weighted images. MR arthrography increases MR sensitivity in detecting TFC tears [45].

There is not a great deal of formal studies about the scapholunate tears in the pediatric population, and for this reason, we cannot use the adult upper limit of 2 mm for the normal width of the space between the two bones until the age of 12 [46].

Distal forearm and scaphoid fractures in children often occur from falls onto an outstretched hand.

Diagnosis is usually achieved by x-ray, but in some cases, it may be difficult to visualize on plain films, although the fracture is present. In fact, occult scaphoid fractures represent 10–15 % of the whole scaphoid lesions. In these cases, MRI may help to identify an occult scaphoid fracture, showing areas of high signal intensity on T2-weighted images, especially in those obtained with short-tau inversion recovery (STIR) (Fig. 6.3) [47].

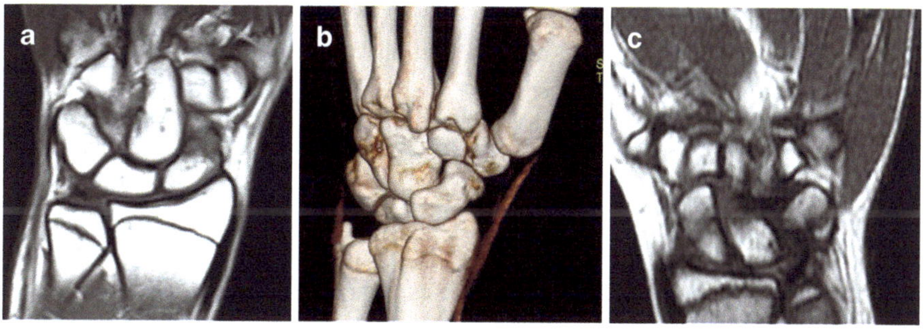

Fig. 6.3 Scaphoid fracture in a 16-year-old-basketball player occurred after a direct blow to the palm. (**a**) T1-weighted image on the coronal plane shows an inhomogeneous aspect of the distal scaphoid pole, characterized by a diffuse area of low signal intensity, with a subtle fracture within it. (**b**) VRT reconstruction on the coronal plane shows the irregular presentation of the distal pole, finding suggestive of fracture. (**c**) Fracture of the body scaphoid, misdiagnosed on plain film in a 10-year-old girl, occurred after a fall onto an outstretched hand. T1-weighted image on coronal plane shows a subtle linear image of low signal intensity at the middle aspect of the bone, suggestive of fracture

US can highlight an irregular aspect of cortical zone which can be misdiagnosed on plain film; it can also show effusion or compartmental hematoma.

Pediatric patients are more likely to suffer from scaphoid tuberosity fracture, which are innocuous unlike scaphoid waist fracture, which may lead to osteonecrosis or nonunion of the proximal pole. Non-displaced waist fracture may appear silent on an initial x-ray; in patients with persistent snuffbox tenderness, MRI can be performed in order to exclude an occult fracture. In this sense, MRI has a 100 % sensitivity for scaphoid fractures, showing a high signal intensity on T2 and a low signal infraction on T1-weighted sequences.

Besides, MRI may also demonstrate marrow edema, and it can also show causes other than fracture, responsible for the patient's pain, such as osseous and soft tissue contusions and capsular-ligament injuries, clinically known as "dorsal wrist pain."

US can be defined as the technique of choice in order to search for ligamentous or tendon lesions.

Gamekeeper's thumb is a common injury in football and basketball players and skiers that occurs following abnormal radially directed force on an abducted thumb. Rupture of the UCL may be total or partial at the distal point of insertion. An avulsion fracture fragment at the ulnar base of the thumb proximal phalanx is typical at the site of UCL attachment. US can show a ligament thickening with an alteration of its normal architecture.

With respect to the contralateral site, it is possible to observe an asymmetrical widening of the first metacarpophalangeal joint on the affected site [48].

MRI is occasionally used to evaluate the soft tissue injury of trigger finger distal avulsion fractures and UCL in patients with a suspected gamekeeper's thumb prior to surgical intervention.

In some UCL tears, we may have the interposition of the adductor aponeurosis between the torn UCL and the bone, a condition known as "Stener lesion," which requires surgical intervention.

Mallet finger occurs when there is an abrupt axial load on a partially flexed finger, and it is characterized by the avulsion of the extensor digitorum tendon from the dorsal aspect of the distal phalanx. This avulsion may be tendinous or, more commonly, go with a small bone fragment of the phalanx. It is easily detectable radiographically [49].

If an avulsion fracture occurs on the volar aspect of the distal phalanx, it is termed "jersey finger," and it develops at the insertion site of the flexor digitorum profundus tendon.

6.2.7 Wrist and Hand: Chronic Injuries

Only a small percentage of young athletes are affected by an overuse condition of the wrist related to wielding rackets, bats, and clubs.

The primary and better known overuse condition of the wrist is the so-called gymnast wrist, more common in female gymnasts, which consists of several conditions affecting the triangular fibrocartilage (TFG) complex tears, interosseous ligament tears, scaphoid stress fractures, ulnar impaction, and ganglion cyst formation.

The repetitive weight bearing on the wrist leads to physeal stress changes of the distal portion of the radius and, sometimes, the ulna. If the injury is stopped, the growth plate may recover itself and the radius may return to normal length; on the contrary, a positive ulnar variance could develop, since the ulna does not undergo the same forces and suffer the same injuries.

The radial physis appears widened, irregular with metaphyseal sclerosis and mild breaking. Later on, the radius appears short due to a delayed growth

MR imaging is more sensitive than x-ray in the detection of physeal changes.

6.3 Lower Limb

6.3.1 Pelvis

Avulsion fractures are common in young athletes aged between 11 and 16 years with a predominance in males.

They usually occur in a "locus minoris resistentiae," represented by the insertion of the tendons at the level of the apophysis that are secondary ossification centers before the fusion. They are mostly composed by cartilage.

Some biomechanical conditions may determine its detachment, such as excessive lengthening or eccentric contraction, especially in subjects with an imbalance of muscle groups.

The biomechanics of these lesions are the same as those in adults, and they are due to a high degree of muscle injuries generally at the myotendinous junction.

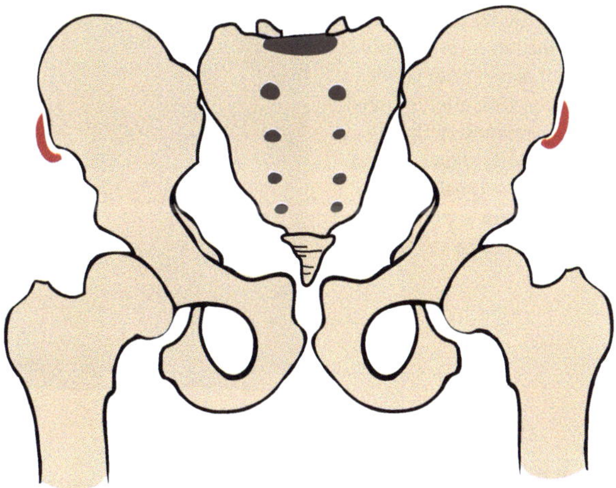

Fig. 6.4 Superior iliac spine (Courtesy of Paola Valori)

X-ray of the pelvis is usually sufficient for the diagnosis and to assess the extent of the lesion.

Ultrasonography is useful when it is difficult to diagnose the radiological extent of the damage in the growth plate.

The sonographic appearance is characterized by an irregular profile, with a modification of the normal echogenicity and a possible hematoma.

MRI examination (and in some cases CT) may be indicated in more complex cases, with the advantage of being able to explore deep parts poorly evaluated by ultrasound.

MRI is a very helpful technique because it can further characterize the injury by showing the bone edema on T2-weighted and STIR images and the focal extension into the unmineralized cartilage [49].

In the bone pelvis, avulsion can occur in different sites [50].

The anterior superior iliac spine is the proximal insertion site of the sartorius and the tensor fascia lata muscle (Fig. 6.4).

Sartorius lesion is common in runners, where athletic effort consists of a forced extension of the hip during knee flexion.

The diagnosis is clinical, but x-ray examination, essential to assess the avulsion extent, can be integrated with a comparative ultrasound examination and with MRI (Fig. 6.5).

The growth plate of the anterior inferior iliac spine appears between 9 and 13 years, welding around 17 years (Fig. 6.6).

At this level, the direct tendon of the anterior rectus muscle of the thigh inserts and its action consists of extending the leg on the thigh and flexing the thigh on the pelvis. The lesion may occur in some sports such as football or rugby, due to a strong contraction against a resistance.

Also in this case, the clinical diagnosis can be integrated with a multidisciplinary study [51–53].

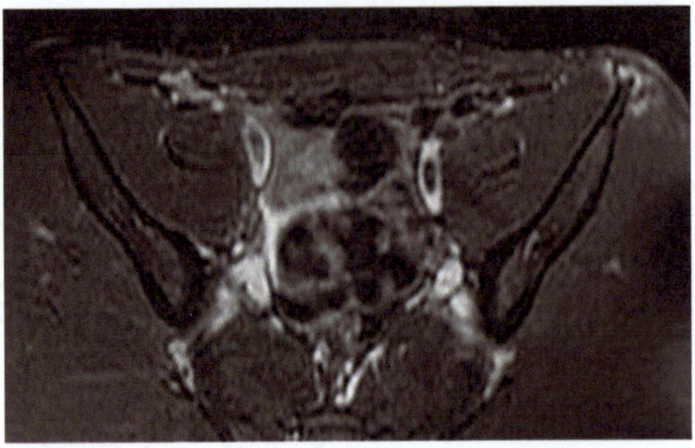

Fig. 6.5 Axial STIR image performed in a 13-year-old football player with pelvic pain occurring after a forced hip hyperextension during running. MRI shows a focal area of high signal intensity of the anterior superior iliac spine, indicating apophysitis

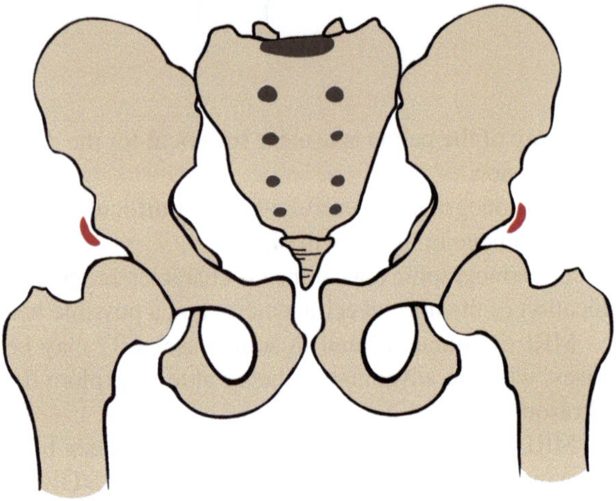

Fig. 6.6 Inferior iliac spine (Courtesy of Paola Valori)

On the other hand, avulsion fractures at the level of the pubic symphysis, where we find the insertion of the adductor muscles, gracilis, and abdominal recti, are rare because they are more often caused by repetitive microtrauma and supported by some anatomical conditions such as asymmetry of the lower limbs [54] (Fig. 6.7).

Ultrasound allows to detect the presence of morphological alterations at the site of tendon insertion.

In these cases, MRI is necessary to study the functional myotendinous unit and bone and cartilaginous components and in particular to search for the "stress response" typically associated with these conditions.

The most common anatomical location of pelvis avulsion fractures is the growth plate of the ischial tuberosity (Fig. 6.8), site of insertion of semimembranosus tendons and hamstrings (composed by semitendinosus and long head of the biceps femoris), characterized by its typical lunate morphology [55] (Fig. 6.9).

The treatment of these injuries is generally conservative, but we have to remember that in some significant (>2 cm) dislocations, the outcome may be disabling.

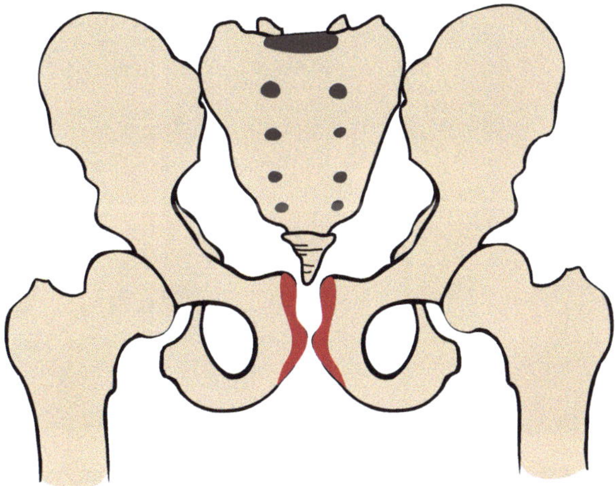

Fig. 6.7 Level of the pubic symphysis (Courtesy of Paola Valori)

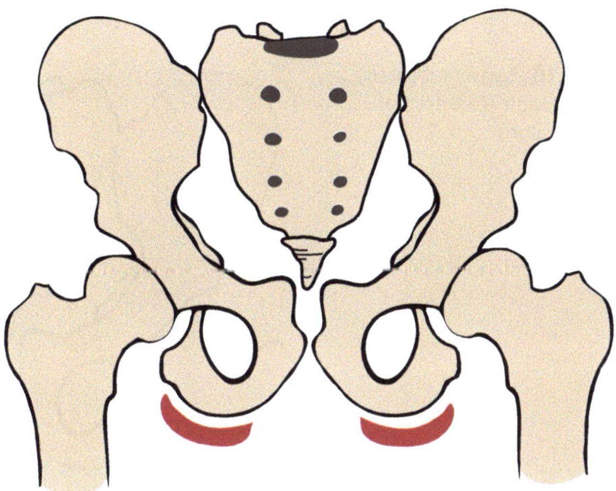

Fig. 6.8 Greater tuberosity (Courtesy of Paola Valori)

MRI is a very useful to assess the degree of soft tissue involvement, to define whether the injury is complete or incomplete, and to assess the relationship with the sciatic nerve.

Avulsions at the iliopsoas insertion on the lesser tuberosity of the femur (Fig. 6.10) or of gluteus or tensor fascia lata muscles at the level of the greater trochanter (Fig. 6.11) are very rare [56].

Legg-Calvè-Perthes disease is a form of idiopathic osteochondrosis of the femoral head physis, rarely connected to overuse injuries, difficult to diagnose both clinically and radiographically.

It occurs early during childhood, generally between 2 and 14 years of age, with a peak around 5–6 years of age, and it is a common cause of pain in children.

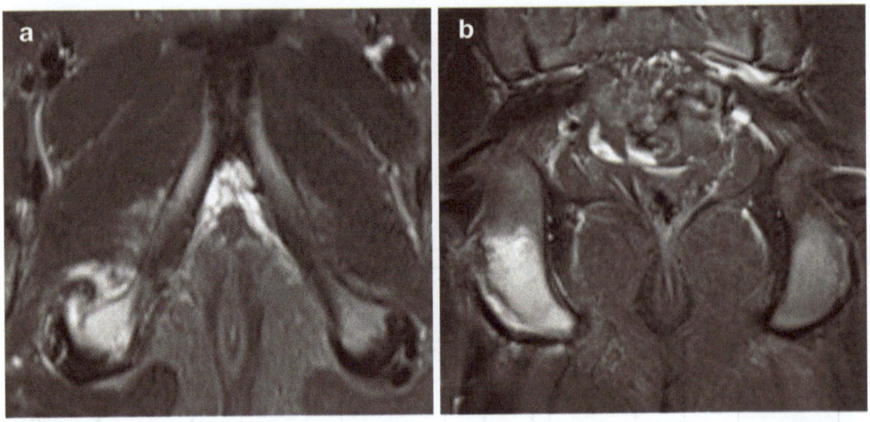

Fig. 6.9 MRI performed in a 12-year-old soccer player. Axial (**a**) and coronal (**b**) STIR images show increased marrow signal of the ischial tuberosity with surrounding periosteal edema and teno-periosteal detachment

Fig. 6.10 Lesser tuberosity of the femur (Courtesy of Paola Valori)

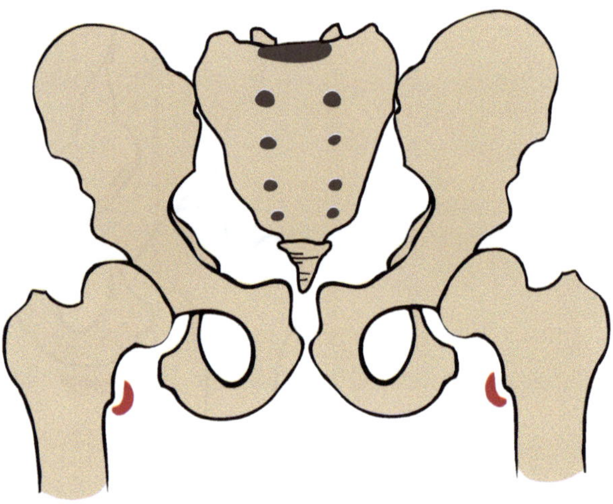

It is usually unilateral, although in 15 % of cases it is bilateral, and it usually affects children between 5 and 8 years old, without a significative history of mechanical abuse.

It is a diagnosis of exclusion, and other causes of avascular necrosis (such as sickle cell disease, leukemia, corticosteroid administration, and Gaucher's disease) as well as epiphyseal dysplasia must be ruled out.

X-ray plays an important role in its diagnosis.

US may be useful just to assess the presence of intra-articular fluid collection [57] (Fig. 6.12).

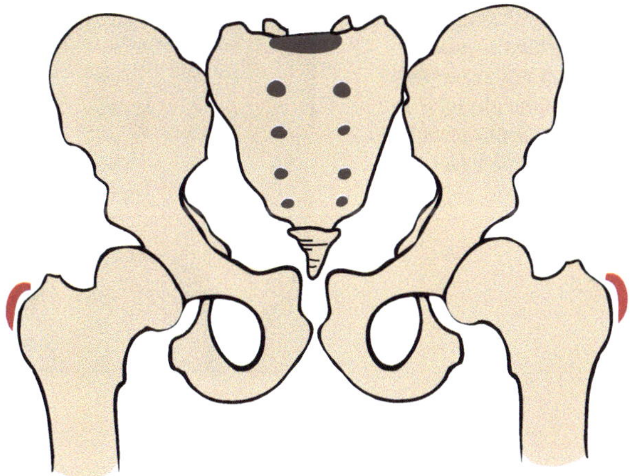

Fig. 6.11 Greater trochanter of the femur (Courtesy of Paola Valori)

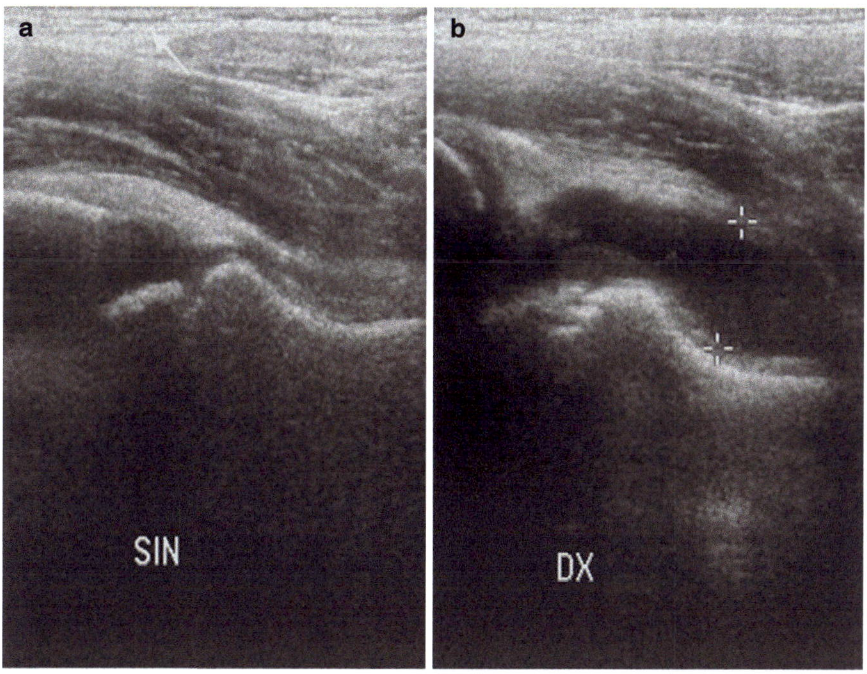

Fig. 6.12 US longitudinal view shows a normal joint (**a**) and the presence of effusion within the left (**b**) joint

MRI may give some essential information to recognize the disease early and to start the therapy as soon as possible; in fact, it has been demonstrated that those children diagnosed at a younger age typically experience a more benign disease

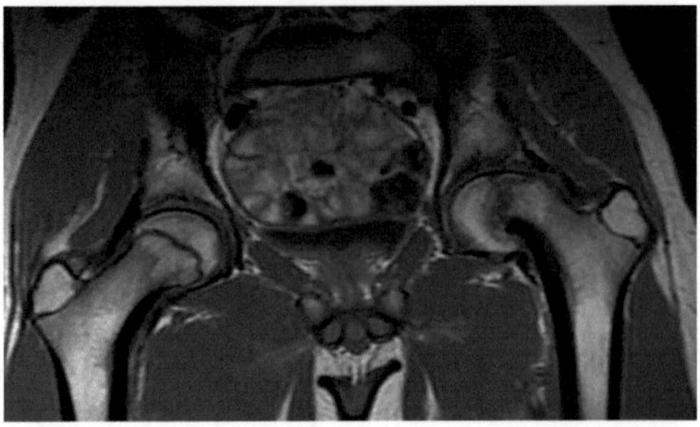

Fig. 6.13 Coronal T1-weighted sequence demonstrates a complete lesion of the physis with posterior displacement and slip of the epiphysis

course, while those diagnosed at an older age typically require increased rates of intervention and generally experience poorer outcomes.

In addition, MRI can accurately stage the disease, evaluate some associated complications, and, above all, differentiate LCP disease from other epiphyseal lesions [58].

Slipped capital femoral epiphysis can result from a chronic overload of compressive and tangential strains acting on the physeal plate, leading to an incomplete or complete lesion, such as type I Salter-Harris lesion. When a complete lesion of the physis occurs, the epiphysis displaces posteriorly and slips.

It can be a real overuse injury when the physis is normal or a relative overuse injury when a normal overload might be excessive for the physeal plate weakened by adverse hormonal conditions (such as hypogonadism).

The diagnosis is easily made by radiography, although MRI can show the "pre-slippage" in controversial cases. It can also highlight edematous changes in the epiphysis and the adjacent metaphysis, and it can also recognize its complications, such as AVN or chondrolysis [59] (Fig. 6.13).

6.3.2 Knee

The knee joint is anatomically made up of the tibiofemoral and the patellofemoral joint.

Capsular-ligament lesions can vary depending on the biomechanics of the trauma, and they occur more frequently in adolescents during sports activity.

It is essential for the radiologist to recognize and interpret the type of lesion also through knowledge of the biomechanical mechanism.

A proper diagnosis is essential to direct the clinician toward the most suitable treatment.

The *Osgood-Schlatter* syndrome, known for more than a century (1903), is the most known osteochondritis, which occurs in some athletes who practice running and jumping, conditions that cause repeated microtrauma to the tibial tubercle, where the patellar tendon inserts.

This condition, more common in males, is usually bilateral, often asymptomatic.

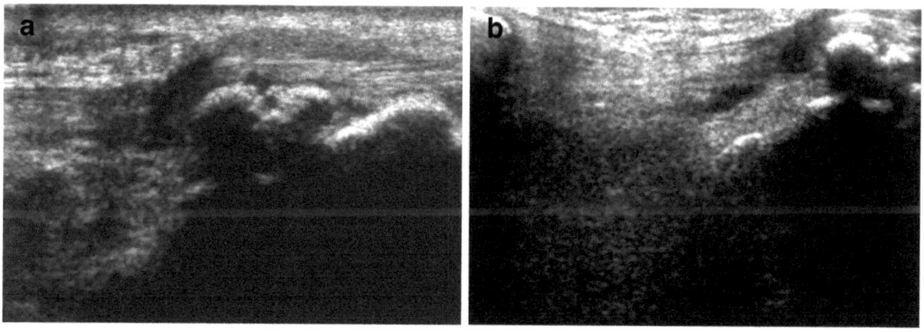

Fig. 6.14 US longitudinal view at the level of the tibial tubercle shows irregularity and fragmentation of the growth plate profile (**a**) thickening of the patellar tendon, and soft tissue swelling (**b**)

The tibial tubercle is an anterior extension of the tibial physis and is prone to injury because of its unique composition, which varies from the other physes.

Since the very beginning, it was described as a pathology affecting firstly the tibial tubercle, but recently, several studies have been demonstrated that the main cause is the action of repetitive microtrauma at the level of tibial insertion of the patellar tendon.

Repetitive stress on the tubercle causes inflammation at the patellar tendon insertion site, reactive bone formation, bone marrow edema, thickening of the proximal portion of patellar tendon, and soft tissue swelling [60, 61].

In addition to the classic findings of bone fragmentation, easily detectable on plain radiographs, ultrasound allows to appreciate the irregularity and fragmentation of the growth plate profile, thickening and abnormal echogenicity of the tendon, and edema of the soft tissue anterior to the tuberosity (Fig. 6.14).

MRI is useful in detecting these signs, especially in the early stage of the disease when only bone marrow edema near the tubercle is visible [62].

This syndrome may predispose to the *avulsion fractures of the tibial tubercle*, in most cases due to a strong knee hyperextension and classified in three types by Watson-Jones, depending on the physis involvement and on the degree of bone fragment dislocation [63].

Sinding-Larsen-Johansson syndrome is a bone avulsion at the proximal patellar insertion.

Ultrasound examination, performed at the patellar inferior pole, highlights the lack of fusion of growth plate of the lower pole of the patella and thickening of the patellar tendon, which appears hypoechoic peripherally, with some rare calcifications.

MRI can determine the extent of the disease, such as fragmentation of the inferior patellar pole, infiltration of Hoffa fat pad, and thickening of the proximal patellar tendon. It is also possible to detect calcification or ossification of the tendon [61, 62].

Isolated rupture of the patellar tendon, generally uncommon in young patients, is usually caused by direct trauma.

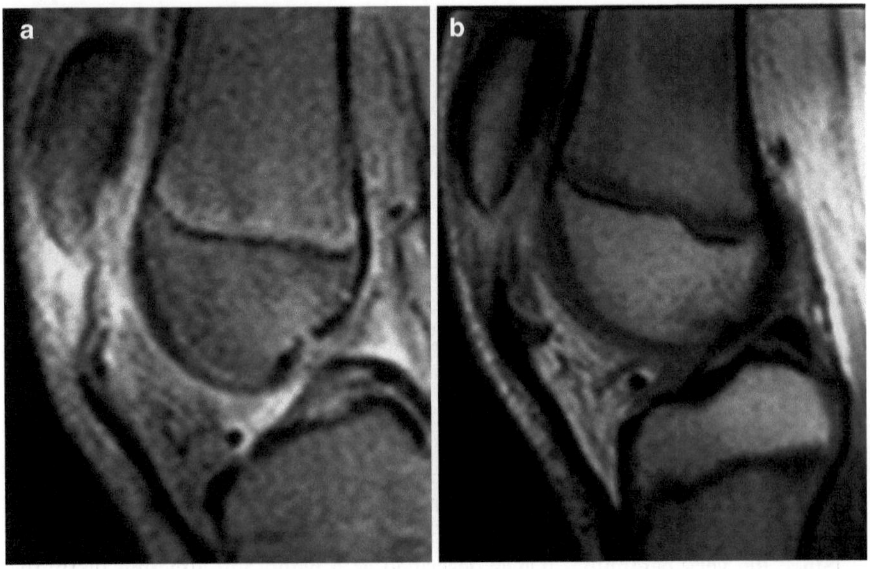

Fig. 6.15 Isolated rupture of the patellar tendon at the level of the distal patellar pole. (**a**, **b**) IR and T1-weighted sequences on sagittal plane show tendon retraction with an inhomogeneous signal intensity and soft tissue swelling

Ultrasound examination allows an accurate assessment of the lesion, with a retracted and hypoechoic appearance of the tendon in the context of a hematoma which can be quantifiable in dimension.

Lateral radiographs can reveal patella alta deformity and one or multiple tiny osseous fragments adjacent to the inferior pole of the patella; in these cases, MRI is indicated for its panoramic views in order to define the exact extent of damage for a possible surgical treatment [64] (Fig. 6.15).

Patellar sleeve avulsion is a cartilaginous injury to the lower pole of the patella.

Conventional radiography is useful in order to define patellar position with respect to the femur and to detect a small bone fragment.

Ultrasonography is useful to search for the cartilage fragment avulsed together with the tendon, but even in these cases, MRI is indicated because it can accurately define the extent of the cartilage damage.

Jumper's knee is a pain syndrome involving the proximal or distal insertion of the patellar tendon, resulting from chronic stress and inflammation, commonly seen in young athletes.

At US examination, the patellar tendon appears hypoechoic in its deep portion with focal loss of the normal fibrillar structure, without signs of hyperemia on power Doppler examination [61].

Other less common conditions are the avulsion of the quadriceps tendon, iliotibial tract, arcuate complex, semimembranosus, or biceps of the femur.

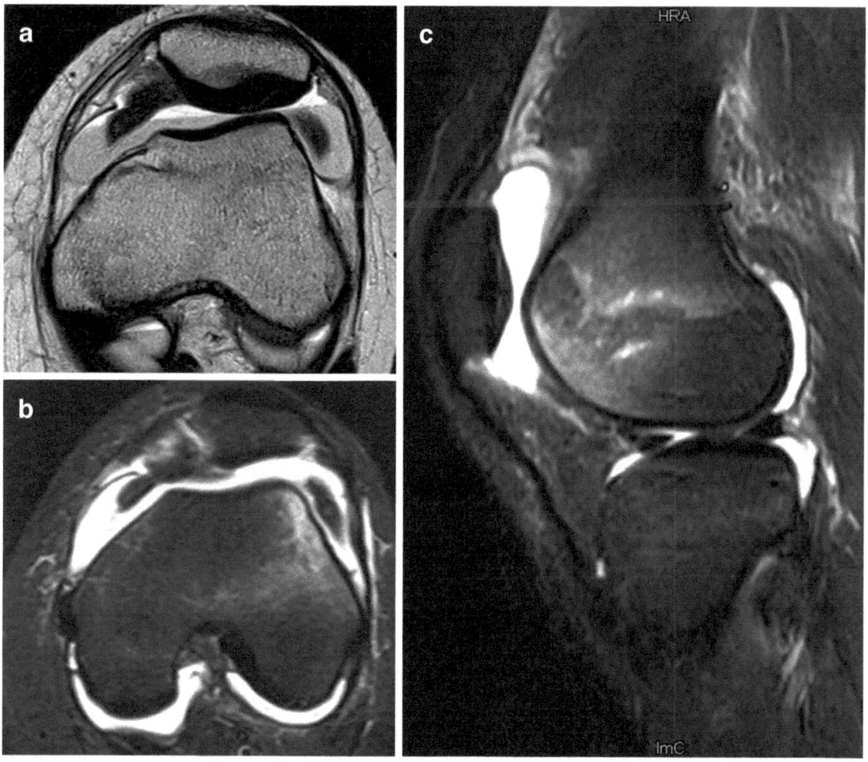

Fig. 6.16 A 15-year-old female patient affected by patella luxation spontaneously reduced. (**a**) T2-weighted image on axial plane shows lipohemarthrosis with three layers visible (from above: fat, fluid, and red blood cells). (**b**, **c**) STIR sequences obtained on the sagittal and axial plane show bone marrow edema on the lateral aspect of the external femoral condyle and on the patella medial aspect, as a consequence of sesamoid luxation

Ultrasound examination is a key contributor in the study of the extensor mechanism, even for anatomical location, and MRI can provide valuable additional information for adequately defining the extent of damage.

Patellofemoral dislocations are acute conditions of loss of normal articular links with sudden lateralization of the sesamoid and distractive injury of the retinacula with a characteristic pattern of injury contusion at the level of the medial articular aspect of the patella and the external condyle of the femur.

These findings are well documented with MRI, which is the test of choice for its diagnosis and also for the evaluation of any dysplastic predisposing conditions and to assess the severity of the ligament damage at the level of the retinacula [63] (Fig. 6.16).

Acute meniscus lesions are more common in adolescents and in those patients with congenital anomaly predisposing morphological variants such as the discoid meniscus.

MRI is definitely crucial to search for meniscus tears (Fig. 6.17).

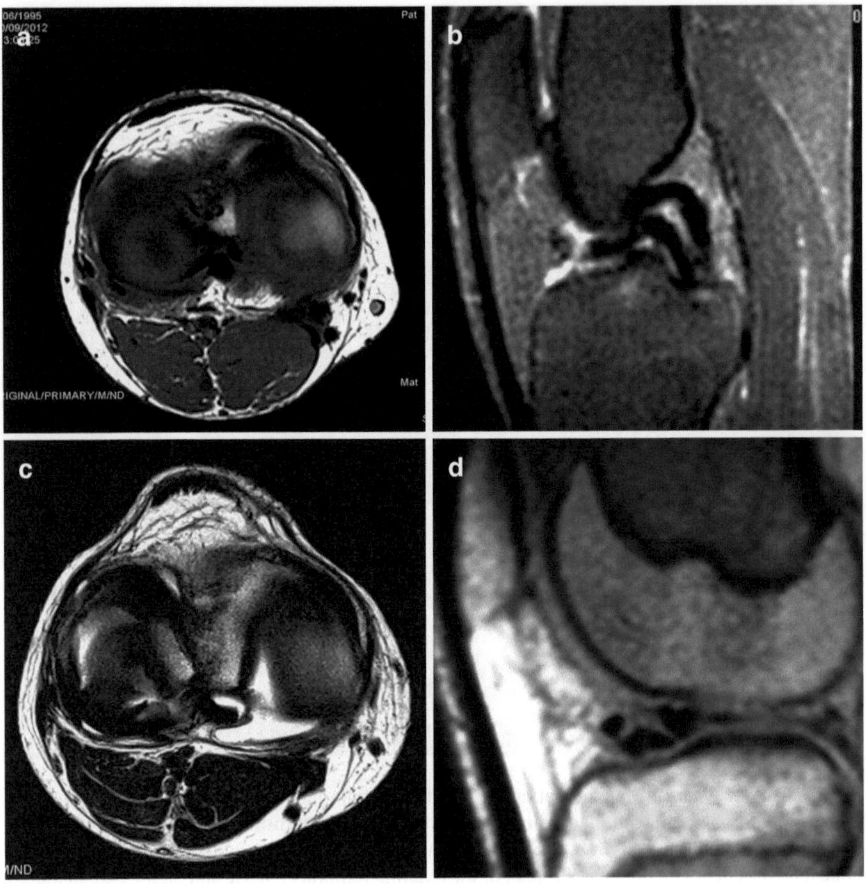

Fig. 6.17 (**a**) A bucket-handle lesion. In the axial plane. (**b**) STIR image on sagittal plane shows the "double posterior cruciate ligament" sign, indicating a bucket-handle lesion. (**c**) Axial plane: lateral meniscus lesion. (**d**) Sagittal plane demonstrates a transverse-oblique lesion of the anterior horn of meniscus

The medial and lateral collateral ligaments are peripheral structures which merge deeply together with the joint capsule and the corresponding corner points, with stabilizing functions complementary to those of the central pivot.

Collateral ligament injuries are well evaluated with ultrasonography, which is a useful tool in determining the degree of injury and the subsequent monitoring.

In partial injury, the ligament appears thickened, hypoechoic and inhomogeneous, but continuous, with rare signs of hyperemia on power Doppler.

In complete injuries, however, the ligament is strongly thickened and hypoechoic, sometimes hardly recognizable and surrounded by fluid collection.

MRI allows to accurately define the degree of injury and the presence of bone bruise and to look for other associated injuries [65] (Fig. 6.18).

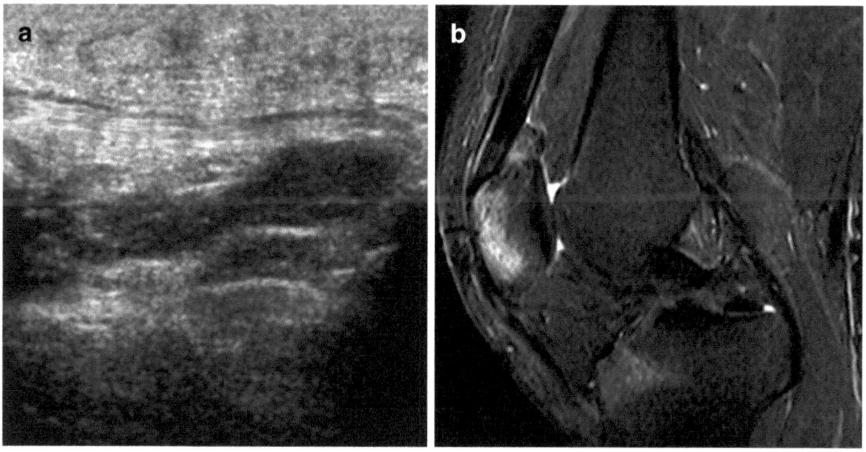

Fig. 6.18 (**a**) US longitudinal view highlights the presence of soft tissue edema and fat-pad congestion. (**b**) STIR sagittal sequence shows marrow edema of the anterior aspect of the patella

Clip pattern lesion is a contact injury that occurs after a pure valgus stress is applied to the knee while the knee is in a state of mild flexion.

It is common among American football players. In this type of lesions, bone marrow edema is usually most prominent in the lateral femoral condyle secondary to direct blow, whereas a second smaller area of edema may be present in the medial femoral condyle secondary to avulsive stress to the MCL.

The main constituents of the central pivot are the cruciate ligaments, intra-articular structures surrounded by the synovial membrane, which are essential to the stability and to the correct functioning of the joint. They are distinct anteriorly and posteriorly according to their anatomical arrangement and insertion on the tibial plate. The lesions are rare in preadolescents and more frequent in sportive adolescents.

The most frequent injuries are those involving the anterior cruciate, easily detected by MRI through assessment of direct and indirect signs.

These lesions are classified according to the site and degree: focal, partial, and complete.

It is also possible to distinguish the phase of injury as acute, subacute, or chronic.

Among the direct signs to look for, the so-called bone contusions (bone bruises) should be taken into consideration.

These findings were considered infrequent in children, but the increasing number of injuries and the number of MRI examinations in young adolescent have modified these concepts.

The distribution and morphology of the contusion areas is a real track of the natural biomechanics of the trauma that helps us to identify the various capsular ligamentous injuries associated with it.

At MRI examination, the contusion lesions appear as areas of low signal intensity on T1-weighted sequences and strongly hyperintense on T2-weighted and STIR sequences.

Pivot shift injury is a noncontact injury commonly seen in skiers or American football players. It occurs when a valgus load is applied to the knee in various states of flexion combined with external rotation of the tibia or internal rotation of the femur. The resulting bone contusion pattern involves the posterior aspect of the lateral tibial plateau and the midportion of the lateral femoral condyle near the condylepatellar sulcus [66, 67].

Hyperextension of the knee can result when direct force is applied to the anterior tibia while the foot is planted or from an indirect force, such as a forceful kicking motion.

It is characterized by edema of the anterior aspect of the condyle and the tibial plate.

Segond avulsion fracture, originally described by the French surgeon Paul Segond in 1879 after a series of cadaveric experiments, involves cortical avulsion of the tibial insertion of the middle third of the lateral capsular ligament.

The mechanism of this injury is often the result of internal rotation of the knee and varus stress, producing abnormal tension on the central portion of the lateral capsular ligament [68, 69].

The lesion consists of an elliptic fragment of bone parallel to the tibia, just distal to the lateral tibial plateau, well detectable on plain radiograph.

Radiographic appearance of Segond fracture is a strong indication for an MRI examination.

MR imaging should be performed in all cases of Segond fracture due to the extensively documented association of this injury with the disruption of the anterior cruciate ligament and meniscal tear.

The Meyers and McKeever classification system describes four degrees of of tibial eminence fractures, and gravity. Tibial eminence fractures are most commonly seen in children and adolescents aged 8 to 14 years depends on the degree of bone fragment dislocation. It usually occurs in children aged between 8 and 14 years.

The first degree is treated conservatively.

The "kissing" bone contusion is a common finding.

The diagnosis must be accurate since the choice of treatment is affected by the degree of injury, the presence of any associated meniscal tears, and especially the degree of skeletal maturity.

Posterior cruciate ligament injury is uncommon in adolescents, and it is typically caused by a direct trauma on the anterior aspect of the tibia when the knee is in a flexed position, as occurs in the *dashboard injury* when the knee strikes against the dashboard during an automobile accident, with a posterior dislocation of the tibia with respect to the femur.

MRI examination will show edema at the anterior aspect of the tibia and, occasionally, at the posterior surface of the patella.

Reverse Segond lesion, recently described, consists of the presence of a bone fragment arising from the medial aspect of the proximal tibia, and it is associated with both midsubstance tears of the posterior cruciate ligament and avulsions of the PCL from the posterior tibial plateau, as well as tears of the medial meniscus.

Osteochondrosis is generally due to a repeated compressive trauma which causes an abnormal blood supply in the stressed area, leading to bone necrosis.

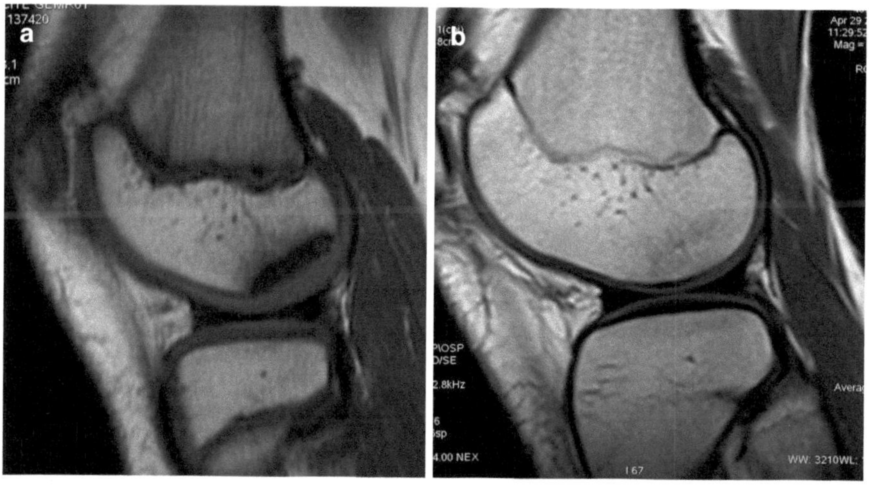

Fig. 6.19 MRI on sagittal plane before and after conservative treatment. (**a**) A diffuse cartilage thickening with a lunate subchondral suffering area on the lateral aspect of the femoral condyle, without cartilage lesion, is evident. (**b**) MRI examination performed after 5 years shows a complete restoration of bone integrity

This alteration generally affects the physeal growth plates, and in younger patients, where the growth plate is in training, the normal process of ossification is compromised until a final deformation.

In young patients, the vascular changes may result in a circumscribed area of osteonecrosis with possible subsequent detachment of a necrotic fragment.

It is important to recognize this condition promptly to establish the most appropriate therapy for the reduction of the overload.

X-ray examination accurately depicts this alteration, especially in an advanced stage. Nevertheless, MRI is the technique of choice which allows to highlight, since the beginning, the deformation of the cortex profile and the evidence of the osteochondral fragment (Fig. 6.19).

Koenig disease is an osteochondral defect of the knee accounting for 80–85 % of all osteochondral lesions. It commonly affects male patients (especially those with florid physis) on the medial femoral condylar epiphysis, as a consequence of repeated microtrauma during athletic activities (Fig. 6.20).

6.3.3 Ankle

Among the most frequent ligament injuries affecting children and adolescents, lesions of ankle inversion trauma with involvement of the external collateral ligament, such as the peroneal-talar component, should be cited. X-ray, allowing to highlight the presence of a fracture or bone detachment, can be integrated with

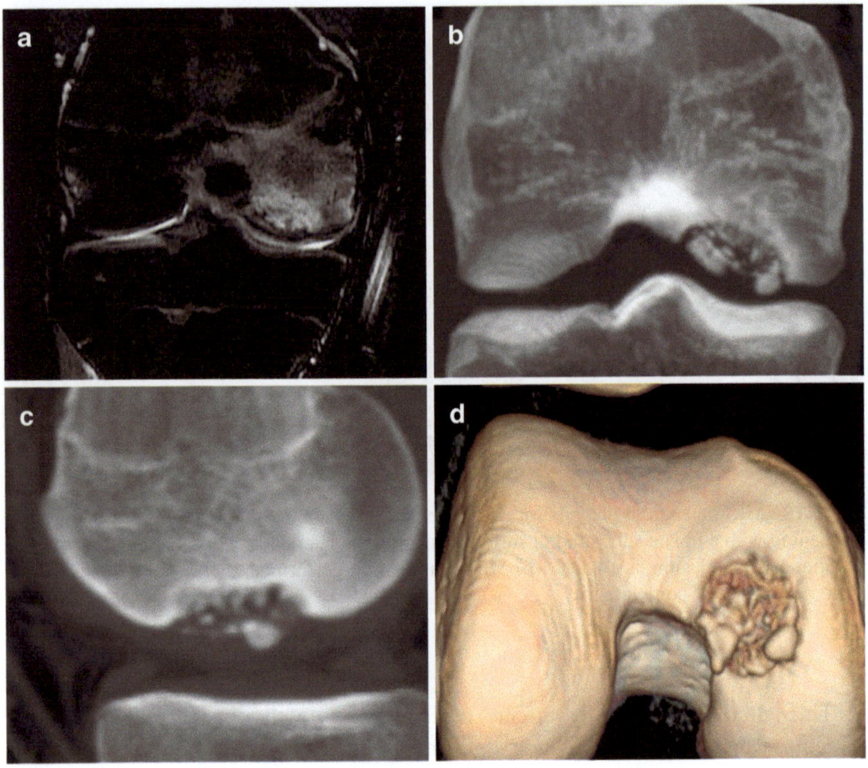

Fig. 6.20 An 8-year-old male patient affected by Koenig disease. (**a**) STIR sequence on the coronal plane shows a subchondral area of marrow edema involving both the articular cartilage and the lateral aspect of the internal femoral condyle, typical signs of osteochondritis. (**b–d**) Coronal, sagittal, and VRT CT reconstructions demonstrate irregularity and fragmentation of the articular cartilage of the internal femoral condyle

ultrasound examination that can show the degree of ligament injury, capsular distension, and the presence of effusion.

MRI provides more information about the evaluation of cartilage components, and it is indicated in high-degree lesions associated with instability [70, 71] (Fig. 6.21).

Osteochondritis dissecans of the talus is a very common disease in running and jumping sports, because of repeated compressive microtrauma. The most common site of lesion is the posterior and internal aspect of the talus. In this case, MRI is a very useful tool in detecting the classical signs of this pathology [71] (Fig. 6.22).

Sever disease is an alteration of the physis plate of the heel, typical of growth age. The most accepted cause is the overloaded performed by the Achilles tendon on heel apophysis. The imaging features are quite similar to those described before, although the radiographic pattern might be confused with a normal densification of apophyseal plate; so, in such difficult cases, MRI can be a reliable tool to make the correct diagnosis [72].

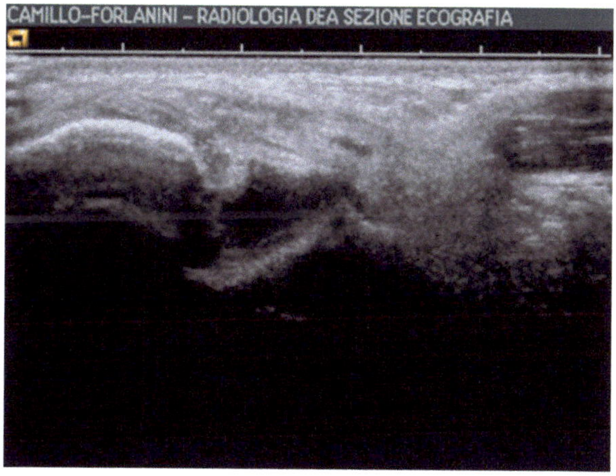

Fig. 6.21 US shows tear of the peroneal-talar component of LCE

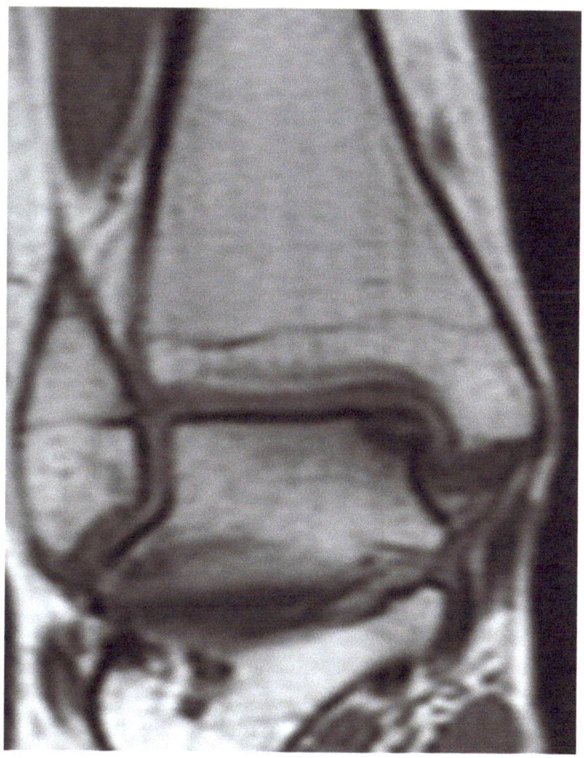

Fig. 6.22 Coronal T1-weighted image shows a lunate hypointense lesion located in the superior aspect of the talus, suggestive of osteochondritis dissecans

It must be stressed that ultrasound examination is very helpful in the differential diagnosis with acute Achilles tendonitis, for the evaluation of peroneal tendons and their anatomical position, and also to evaluate the posterior tibial tendon and the common flexor and extensor compartment.

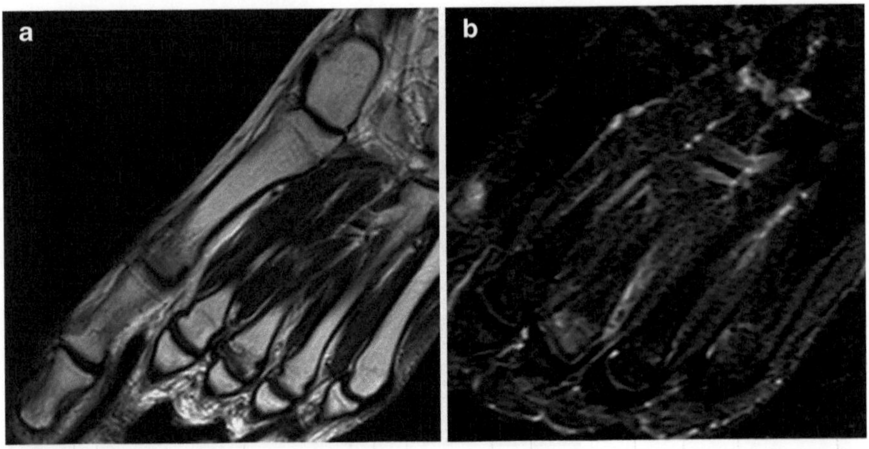

Fig. 6.23 MRI coronal oblique (**a**–**b**) plains show signal alteration on the third metatarsal head, suggestive of Freiberg disease

Iselin disease is an osteochondrosis of the fifth metatarsal base, caused by a traction mechanism of the peroneal tendons.

Freiberg disease affects the physeal plate of the second metatarsal head and, rarely, the third, and it commonly occurs in runner athletes. MRI can be useful in the evaluation of spongeous bone which appears hyperintense on T2-weighted images, indicating bone marrow edema [73] (Fig. 6.23).

6.4 Acute Stress Injuries in Children

Stress fractures are acute injuries caused by repetitive microtrauma during sports activity. These conditions are common in practicing athletics.

Typical locations of stress fractures are the tibia, fibula, femur, tarsal, and metatarsal bones.

They clinically present with swelling and pain related to physical activity, without a history of acute injury.

They are not easily detected with conventional radiography, especially in the acute setting when the examination is driven by painful symptoms, and cortical thickening and spongeous reaction are not visible.

In acute phase, MRI is the best diagnostic modality, owing to its high sensitivity in detecting marrow edema, which results in low signal intensity on T1-weighted images and high signal intensity on STIR and T2-weighted images. The fracture line, on the other hand, is well depicted as a low signal intensity on both T1- and T2-weighted sequences (Fig. 6.24).

Subperiosteal fluid is a helpful ancillary finding in a subtle fracture.

Immature skeleton is particularly prone to stress injuries; this is due to some factors, such as increased physical activities, narrower bones with thinner cortices, hormonal changes, and less muscle mass.

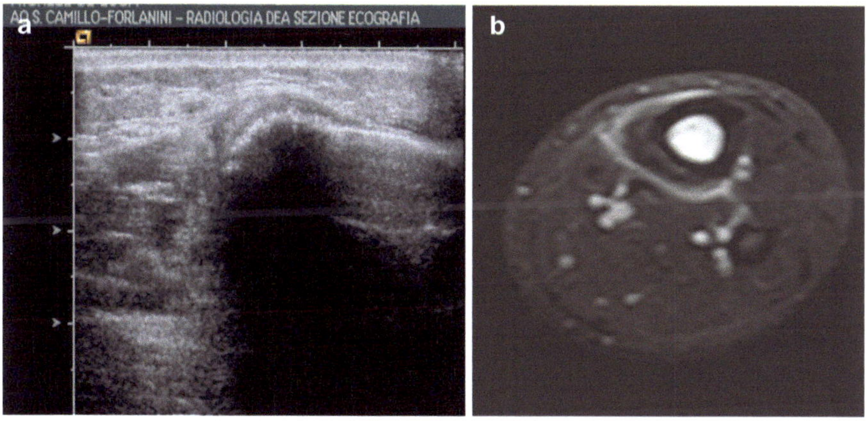

Fig. 6.24 A 17-year-old runner suffering from edema and tenderness of the right leg. (**a**) US shows soft tissue swelling. (**b**) Axial STIR sequence shows signal alteration characterized by a diffuse area of high signal intensity, suggestive of marrow edema

Stress injuries can occur in a healthy bone which undergo a functional overuse cyclically repeated, which causes microscopic injuries that, when frequently *applied*, do not allow a complete structural restoration, leading to anatomical alterations and particular clinical features.

In fact, when a bone is subject to stress, initially it responds with an accelerated cortical resorption and remodeling of the haversian system, inducing a cortex weakening; a prolonged stress results in osteoclastic resorption outpacing osteoblastic repair, causing even further weakening and fracture if the stressor is not reduced.

These lesions, less common in adult patients, are the leading cause of sports injuries in young athletes, maybe because during growth, sudden changes in body size could complicate the coordination of athletic movements, thus modifying the strain type and, therefore, increasing the chance of stress injuries.

In the physis, long-standing overuse affects the endochondral ossification, resulting in abnormal physeal widening and, occasionally, bone bridging [74].

Toddler's stress fractures of the lower extremities are associated with the onset of ambulation. They typically occur between 9 months and 3 years of age, and they manifest with a refusal to bear weight and are not preceded by a recognized acute traumatic event.

The typical toddler's fracture is a non-displaced oblique fracture of the distal portion of the tibia. Other locations are the fibula, the posterior aspect of the calcaneus, the talus, and the base of the cuboid.

Stress fractures of the pelvic bones are difficult to detect radiographically owing to its anatomical complexity and bowel gas interposition.

The most common bones involved are the pubis and the sacrum; they usually affect young runners and sometimes volleyball players and gymnasts.

Stress fractures of the upper extremities are less common, where the ulna and radius are the most frequently involved bones, especially in tennis players, and the olecranon apophysis in gymnasts. Stress fractures of the carpal bones are uncommon in young patients, and they often are underdiagnosed. The capitate is the most frequently affected bone, followed by lunate and scaphoid.

The lumbar spine and sacral spine are common sites of stress fractures observed during the teenage growth spurt, and they involve the pars interarticularis, causing spondylolysis, with or without spondylolisthesis.

It usually occurs before 16 years as a gradual vertebral slip, but the patient is typically asymptomatic.

This condition has been encountered in as many as 47 % of adolescent athletes with low back pain, with respect to only 5 % of adult athletes with the same symptom.

Stress injuries of the pars interarticularis range from changes in signal intensity, such as stress response, to bony defects. The prognosis is worse when there is nonunion.

6.5 Muscle Lesions

Muscle derangements in athletes have a wide variety of causes, treatments, and prognoses.

They represent 10–30 % of all sports injuries in young adolescents, and they require an accurate diagnosis because the therapeutic treatment is based on a correct clinical reading of the lesions.

They usually occur at the onset of athletic activity, involving more frequently the lower limb muscles crossing two joints, such as the rectus femoris, hamstrings, and gastrocnemius muscles. They commonly affect the myotendinous junction but sometimes also the muscular belly.

There are some predisposing factors such as fatigue, outside temperature, electrolyte imbalances, poor training, recovery after long injury, "recovery of athletic preparation," and one of the considerable impacts, the "imbalance" between agonistic and antagonistic muscle groups.

Their incidence gradually increases in the last phase of adolescence, owing to a gradual strengthening of tendinous junctions, shifting the site of minor resistance toward the muscle.

The clinical impact of diagnostic imaging is very significant owing to the fact that its classification, necessary to assess the degree of injury, to direct the treatment, and to define the recovery time, is based on clinical and radiological criteria.

Given that the cause and severity of athletic injuries may be difficult to determine clinically, US and MR imaging are utilized increasingly to evaluate muscle injuries, especially in young athletes.

Ultrasonography is the first-choice technique in the acute setting, since it has a high cost-benefit ratio, is easily repeatable and therefore useful in the monitoring of the lesions, and is well tolerated by the patient.

It is also possible to evaluate the dynamics of muscle in comparison with the contralateral side.

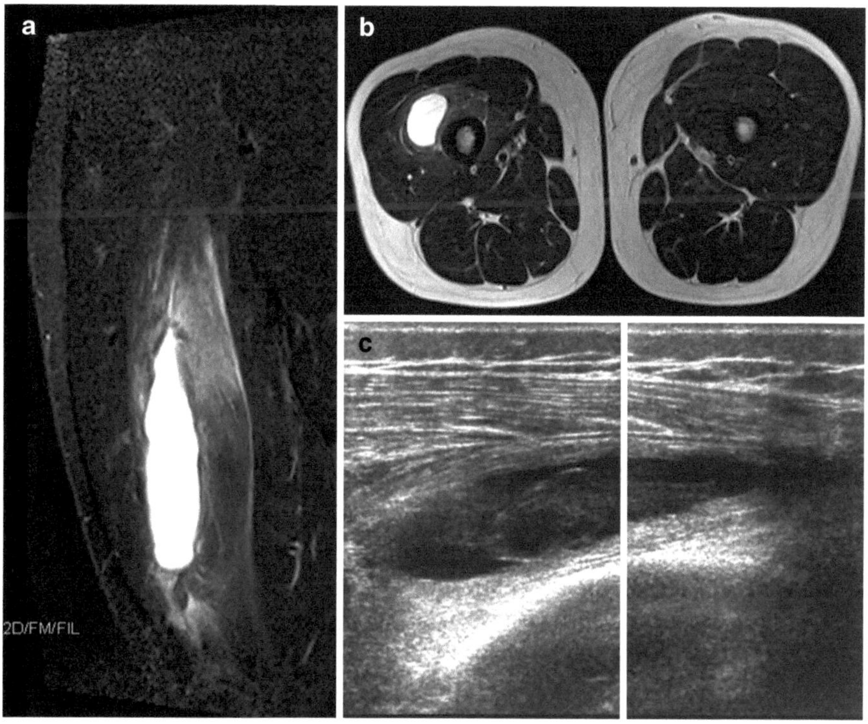

Fig. 6.25 (**a**, **b**) Wide area of high signal intensity on STIR image within the lateral aspect of the femur quadriceps. (**c**) US performed on the corresponding area shows a large intramuscular hematoma

MRI is highly sensitive in the diagnosis of low-grade lesions owing to its high contrast resolution, its multiplanarity, and its ability to explore the deep layers [75].

In some traumatic conditions, when clinical findings are subtle or absent, MR imaging becomes essential to reach the correct diagnosis (Fig. 6.25).

Muscle lesions can be divided, depending on the cause of the trauma, into direct (such as contusions) and indirect injuries.

Muscle contusions are the most common type of muscle injuries occurring during the pediatric age, particularly in the first adolescence, and they usually involve lower limb muscles (quadriceps and tibialis anterior) exhibiting pain, swelling, ecchymosis, spasm, and functional limitation.

MR imaging is quite similar to that of indirect injuries, although the site usually is deep, adjacent to the bone surface, owing to the different traumatic cause.

Muscle girth is usually increased, without fiber discontinuity or laxity.

On T2-weighted sequences, a large area of high signal intensity, with a diffuse or geographic appearance, may be displayed, often with feathery margins. In such hard cases, the edema is associated to a muscular hematoma.

Indirect injuries are muscle strains due to the application of longitudinal forces overcoming the elastic strength of muscular fibers.

They are classified using a three-grade continuous spectrum of injury, from mild (first degree) to severe (third degree), and low-grade injuries are more common than high-grade ones.

A mild lesion is characterized by microscopic injury to the muscle or tendon.

The treatment is conservative, consisting in rest from aggravating activities.

A moderate lesion (partial-thickness tear) consists of a tissue damage involving 2/3 of the muscle belly, and it exhibits a sudden, acute and localized pain associated with function limitation.

A severe lesion (complete disruption), typically at the site of junction, involves the whole muscular section, with or without retraction; it exhibits with strong pain and a complete loss of muscular function. Sometimes, it requires surgical intervention.

Grading the tears by US:

- Mild lesion (first degree – elongation): US can be negative or can show the presence of a small hypoechoic area within the muscular fibers. Healing is quick, usually in 15 days.
- Moderate lesion (second degree): in the acute setting (<24 h), we can find the presence of a hyperechoic hematoma which often underestimates the underlying muscle injury. It appears as a discontinuity of the muscular fibrolipidic septa, with some hypo-anechoic areas with irregular edges.
- Severe lesion (third degree): complete breakdown of muscle fibers resulting in mass effect associated with distal muscle fiber retraction and adjacent effusion.

Grading the tears by MRI [76]:

- Grade I tear: focal high signal intensity on T2-weighted and STIR sequences with muscle edema and hemorrhage at the myotendinous junction; edema and hemorrhage may track along muscle fascicles, creating a feathery margin to the lesion. We can also find a rim of hyperintense perifascial fluid around a muscle belly or a group of muscles.
- Grade II tear: this is a partial-thickness strain of the myotendinous junction with interstitial feathery high signal intensity on T2-weighted sequences or hematoma in the acute setting. Perifascial fluid also is common in this situation. Low signal can represent either fibrosis or hemosiderin and can be seen in chronic or old injuries.
- Grade III tear: it represents a complete myotendinous disruption, and if muscle retraction is associated, it can be seen as an enlargement of the retracted belly with a focal fluid collection filling the gap. It is also associated with a significant hematoma formation.

Some complications of muscle injuries include myositis ossificans and rarely compartment syndrome or pyomyositis.

At US examination, the posttraumatic scarring alterations may appear as hyperechoic linear streaks after an indirect distractive trauma or as nodular areas with streaks of increased echogenicity after a blunt trauma.

Muscle laceration is caused by a penetrating injury and is uncommon in athletic patients. MR imaging is not usually performed in the acute setting, although it may show a focal and sharp discontinuity of fibers and a high signal intensity on T2-weighted sequences, caused by hemorrhage and edema.

Muscle herniation refers to the protrusion of muscle belly through a focal fascia defect (such as those traversed by vessels and nerves) caused, in traumatic setting, by a tear, a penetrating lesion, or fractures; more commonly, it usually occurs because of muscle hypertrophy and increased intracompartmental pressure.

The most involved sites are the middle to the lower portions of the leg, with the tibialis anterior most commonly involved.

MR imaging shows an outward muscle bulging with a discontinuity in the overlying fascia.

References

1. Kumar R, Lindell MM, Madewell JE et al (1989) The clavicle: normal and abnormal. Radiographics 9(4):677–706
2. Curtis RJJ (1994) Skeletal injuries: shoulder injuries. In: Stanitski CL, DeLee JC, Drez D (eds) Pediatric and adolescent sports medicine. W.B. Saunders, Philadelphia, pp 175–215
3. Cleeman E, Flatow EL (2000) Shoulder dislocations in the young patient. Orthop Clin North Am 31(2):217–229
4. Rowe CR (1956) Prognosis in dislocations of the shoulder. J Bone Joint Surg Am 38-A(5):957–977
5. Emery KH (2006) Imaging of sports injuries of the upper extremity in children. Clin Sports Med 25:513–568
6. Deitch J, Menhlman CT, Food SL et al (2003) Traumatic anterior shoulder dislocation in adolescents. Am J Sports Med 31(5):758–763
7. Marans HJ, Angel KR, Schemitsch EH et al (1992) The fate of traumatic anterior dislocation of the shoulder in children. J Bone Joint Surg Am 74(8):1242–1244
8. Magee T, Williams D, Mani N (2004) Shoulder MR arthrography: which patient group benefits most? AJR Am J Roentgenol 183(4):969–974
9. Meister K, Thesing J, Montgomery WJ et al (2004) MR arthrography of partial thickness tears of the undersurface of the rotator cuff: an arthroscopic correlation. Skeletal Radiol 33(3): 136–141
10. Lee SY, Lee JK (2002) Horizontal component of partial thickness tears of rotator cuff: imaging characteristics and comparison of ABER view with oblique coronal view at MR arthrography initial results. Radiology 224(2):470–476
11. Bui Mansfield LT, Banks KP, Taylor DC (2007) Humeral avulsion of the glenohumeral ligaments: the HAGL lesion. Am J Sports Med 35:1960–1966
12. Dahlin LB, Erichs K, Andersson C et al (2007) Incidence of early posterior shoulder dislocation in brachial plexus birth palsy. J Brachial Plex Peripher Nerve Inj 2:24
13. Tung GA, Hou DD (2003) MR arthrography of the posterior labrocapsular complex: relationship with glenohumeral joint alignment and clinical posterior instability. AJR Am J Roentgenol 180:369–375
14. Bradley JP, Baker CL 3rd, Kline AJ et al (2006) Arthroscopic capsulolabral reconstruction for posterior instability of the shoulder: a prospective study of 100 shoulder. Am J Sports Med 34:1061–1071
15. May MM, Bishop K (2013) Shoulder injuries in young athletes. Pediatr Radiol 43:135–140
16. Heyworth BE, Williams RJ 3rd (2009) Internal impingement of the shoulder. Am J Sports Med 37:1024–1037

17. Kanati U, Ozturk BY, Bolukbasi S (2010) Anatomical variations of the anterosuperior labrum: prevalence and association with type II superior labrum anterior-posterior (SLAP) lesions. J Shoulder Elbow Surg 19:1199–1203
18. Piatt BE, Hawkins RJ, Fritz RC et al (2002) Clinical evaluation and treatment of spinoglenoid notch ganglion cysts. J Shoulder Elbow Surg 11:600–604
19. Chen FS, Diaz VA, Loebenberg M et al (2005) Shoulder and elbow injuries in the skeletally immature athlete. J Am Acad Orthop Surg 13(3):172–185
20. Carson WG Jr, Grasser SI (1998) Little Leaguer's shoulder. A report of 23 cases. Am J Sports Med 26(4):575–580
21. Song JC, Lazarus ML, Song AP (2006) MRI findings in Little Leaguer's shoulder. Skeletal Radiol 35(2):107–109
22. Wasserlauf BL, Paletta GA Jr (2003) Shoulder disorders in the skeletally immature throwing athlete. Orthop Clin North Am 34(3):427–437
23. Paley KJ, Jobe FW, Pink MM et al (2000) Arthroscopic findings in the overhead throwing athlete: evidence for posterior internal impingement of the rotator cuff. Arthroscopy 16(1):35–40
24. Sanders TG, Miller MD (2005) A systematic approach to magnetic resonance imaging interpretation of sports medicine injuries of the shoulder. Am J Sports Med 33(7):1088–1105
25. Vinson EN, Helms CA, Higgins LD (2007) Rim-rent tear of the rotator cuff: a common and easily overlooked partial tear. AJR Am J Roentgenol 189(4):943–946
26. Giaroli EL, Major NM, Higgins LD (2005) MRI of internal impingement of the shoulder. AJR Am J Roentgenol 185(4):925–929
27. Beltran J, Rosenberg ZS (1997) MR imaging of pediatric elbow fractures. Magn Reson Imaging Clin N Am 5(3):567–578
28. Carey J, Spence L, Blickman H et al (1998) MRI of pediatric growth plate injury: correlation with plain film radiographs and clinical outcome. Skeletal Radiol 27(5):250–255
29. Major NM, Crawford ST (2002) Elbow effusion in trauma in adults and children: is there an occult fracture? AJR Am J Roentgenol 178:413–418
30. White PG, Mah JY, Friedman L (1994) Magnetic resonance imaging in acute physeal injuries. Skeletal Radiol 23:527
31. Lyman S, Fleisig GS, Andrews JR, Osinski ED (2002) Effect of pitch type, pitch count, and pitching mechanics on risk of elbow and shoulder pain in youth baseball pitchers. Am J Sports Med 30(4):463–468
32. Kijowsku R, Tuite MJ (2010) Pediatric throwing injuries of the elbow. Semin Musculoskelet Radiol 14(4):419–429
33. Greiwe RM, Saifi C, Ahmad CS (2010) Pediatric sports elbow injuries. Clin Sports Med 29(4):677–703
34. Rudzki JR, Paletta GA Jr (2004) Juvenile and adolescent elbow injuries in sports. Clin Sports Med 23(4):581–608
35. Timmermann LA, Andrews JR (1994) Undersurface tear of the ulnar collateral ligament in baseball players. A newly recognized lesion. Am J Sports Med 22(1):33–36
36. Sugimoto H, Ohsawa T (1994) Ulnar collateral ligament in the growing elbow: MR imaging of normal development and throwing injuries. Radiology 192(2):417–422
37. Hayter CL, Adler RS (2012) Injuries of the elbow and the current treatment of tendon disease. AJR Am J Roentgenol 199:546–557
38. Iyer RS, Thapa MM, Khanna PC et al (2012) Pediatric bone imaging: imaging elbow trauma in children – a review of acute and chronic injuries. AJR Am J Roentgenol 198:1053–1068
39. Benjamin HJ, Briner WW Jr (2005) Little league elbow. Clin J Sport Med 15(1):37–40
40. KijowskuR DSAA (2005) Radiography of the elbow for evaluation of patients with osteochondritis dissecans of the capitellum. Skeletal Radiol 34(5):266–271
41. Kramer J, Stiglbauer R, Engel A, Prayer L, Imhof H (1992) MR contrast arthrography (MRA) in ostechondrosis dissecans. J Comput Assist Tomogr 16(2):254–260
42. Zetaruk MN (2000) The young gymnast. Clin Sports Med 19(4):757–780
43. Kocher MS, Waters PM, Micheli LJ (2000) Upper extremity injuries in the paediatric athlete. Sports Med 30(2):117–135

44. Zlatkin MB, Rosner J (2004) MR imaging of ligaments and triangular fibrocartilage complex of the wrist. Magn Reson Imaging Clin N Am 12:301–331
45. Schweitzer ME, Natale P, Winalski CS, Culp R (2000) Indirect wrist MR arthrography: the effects of passive motion versus active exercise. Skeletal Radiol 29:10–14
46. Kaawach W, Ecklund K, Di Canzio J, Zurakowski D, Waters PM (2001) Normal ranges of scapholunate distance in children 6 to 14 years old. J Pediatr Orthop 21(4):464–467
47. Eustace S, Denison W (1997) Pictorial review: magnetic resonance imaging of acute orthopaedic trauma to the upper extremity. Clin Radiol 52:338–344
48. Gaca AM (2009) Basketball injuries in children. Pediatr Radiol 39(12):1275–1285
49. Pan J, Bredella MA (2013) Imaging of soft tissue abnormalities about the hip. Radiol Clin North Am 51:353–369
50. Stevens MA, El- Khoury GY, Kathol MH et al (1999) Imaging features of avulsion Injuries. Radiographics 19:655–672
51. Bancroft LW, Blankenbaker DG (2010) Imaging of the tendons about the pelvis. AJR Am J Roentgenol 195:605–617
52. Gyftopoulos S, Rosenberg ZS, Schweitzer ME et al (2008) Normal anatomy and strains of the deep musculotendinous junction of the proximal rectus femoris: MRI features. AJR Am J Roentgenol 190:182–186
53. Galloway HR (2013) Overuse injuries of the lower extremity. Radiol Clin North Am 51:511–528
54. Omar IM, Zoga AC, Kavanagh EC et al (2008) Athletic pubalgia and "sports hernia": optimal MR imaging technique and findings. Radiographics 28:1415–1438
55. Koulouris G, Connell D (2003) Evaluation of the hamstring muscle complex following acute injury. Skeletal Radiol 32:582–589
56. Patel K, Wallace R, Busconi BD (2011) Radiology. Clin Sports Med 30:239–283
57. Stuecker MH, Habermann C, Bubenheim M et al (2008) Sonography for evaluation of containment in perthes disease: a comparison with magnetic resonance imaging. Ultraschall Med 29(Suppl 5):245–249
58. Stücker MH, Buthmann J, Meiss AL (2005) Evaluation of hip containment in legg-calvé-perthes disease: a comparison of ultrasound and magnetic resonance imaging. Ultraschall Med 26(5):406–410
59. Harland U, Krappel FA (2002) Value of ultrasound, CT, and MRI in the diagnosis of slipped capital femoral epiphysis (SCFE). Orthopade 31(9):851–856, German
60. Draghi F, Danesino GM, Coscia D et al (2008) Overload syndromes of the knee in adolescents: sonographic findings. J Ultrasound 11(4):151–157
61. Carr JC, Hanly S, Griffin J et al (2001) Sonography of the patellar tendon and adjacent structures in pediatric and adult patients. AJR Am J Roentgenol 176:1535–1539
62. Dupuis CS, Westra SJ, Makris J et al (2009) Injuries and conditions of the extensor mechanism of the pediatric knee. Radiographics 29:877–886
63. Gottsegen CJ, Eyer BA, White EA et al (2008) Avulsion fractures of the knee: imaging findings and clinical significance. Radiographics 28(6):1755–1770
64. Ostlere S (2013) The extensor mechanism of the knee. Radiol Clin North Am 51:393–411
65. Lopomo N, Zaffagnini S, Amis AA (2013) Quantifying the pivot shift test: a systematic review. Knee Surg Sports Traumatol Arthrosc 21(4):767–783
66. Ahldén M, Samuelsson K, Fu FH et al (2013) Rotatory knee laxity. Clin Sports Med 32:37–46
67. Dodds AL, Halewood C, Gupte CM et al (2014) The anterolateral ligament: anatomy, length changes and association with the Segond fracture. Bone Joint J 96-B(3):325–331
68. Geiger D, Chang E, Pathria M et al (2013) Posterolateral and posteromedial corner injuries of the knee. Radiol Clin North Am 51:413–432
69. Vanhoenacker FM, Snoeckx A (2007) Bone marrow edema in sports: general concepts. Eur J Radiol 62:6–15
70. Hunt KJ, Githens M, Riley GM et al (2013) Foot and ankle injuries in sport imaging correlation with arthroscopic and surgical findings. Clin Sports Med 32:525–557

71. Nazarenko A, Beltran LS, Bencardino JT (2013) Imaging evaluation of traumatic ligamentous injuries of the ankle and foot. Radiol Clin North Am 51:455–478
72. Bailey CW, Cannon ML (2014) Sever disease (calcaneal apophysitis). J Am Osteopath Assoc 114(5):411
73. Talusan PG, Diaz-Collado PJ, Reach JS Jr (2014) Freiberg's infraction: diagnosis and treatment. Foot Ankle Spec 7(1):52–56
74. Berger FH, de Jonge MC, Maas M (2007) Stress fractures in the lower extremity. The importance of increasing awareness amongst radiologists. Eur J Radiol 62:16–26
75. May DA, Disler DG, Jones EA et al (2000) Abnormal signal intensity in skeletal muscle at MR imaging: patterns, pearls, and pitfalls. Radiographics 20:S295–S315
76. Elsayes KM, Lammle M, Shariff A et al (2006) Value of magnetic resonance imaging in muscle trauma. Curr Probl Diagn Radiol 35:206–212

7 Diagnostic Imaging in Child Abuse

Domenico Barbuti, Laura Tanturri de Horatio, and Marco Cirillo

Child abuse is an issue of great relevance increasing everywhere in the world. In the United States, 1 % of children suffer from different types of maltreatment, the main forms being neglect (63 % of cases), physical abuse (19 %), sexual abuse (10 %), and psychologic abuse (8 %), with an overall mortality of 1,200/year [1]. Girls are abused slightly more often than boys (12.8 vs 11.2 for girls and boys, respectively, per 1,000 children). Clinical features include bruises; lacerations; scratches; burns or scalds; eye, head, and visceral injuries; boxer's nose; poisoning; suffocation; fractures; and genital and anal injury. Signs of neglect can be also found: lack of hygiene or care, failure to thrive, obesity, vitamin deficit, delayed development, and untreated medical conditions. Abused children present often emotional signs consisting of unhappiness, anger, low self-esteem, anxiety, depression or suicidal mania, and unexplained symptoms of illness. The consequences of abuse can be serious and longstanding; in case of brain injury, permanent handicap or even death may occur. The first description of child abuse was made by Tardieu [2] in 1860. In 1946, Caffey [3] described six infants with subdural hematomas and long-bone fractures in his opinion following abuse, and later described as metaphyseal fracture which are considered to date the most specific injury in child abuse [4]. In 1962, Kempe et al. coined the term *battered child syndrome* to describe metaphyseal fracture and other injuries typical of abuse [5]. In 1971, Guthkelch [6] invoked shaking (shaken baby syndrome) as the causative mechanism in abusive head injury. Kleinman contributed to understand the pathophysiology and mechanisms of injury in non-accidental trauma [7]. Actually "non-accidental injury (NAI)" is mostly employed to define this condition.

Imaging plays an important role in the detection and documentation of NAI, differentiating abuse from accidental trauma, normal variants, metabolic bone diseases, and skeletal dysplasias. Failure of a correct diagnosis may have serious

D. Barbuti, MD (✉) • L. Tanturri de Horatio, MD • M. Cirillo, MD
Department of Diagnostic Imaging, Bambino Gesù Children's Hospital IRCCS, Rome, Italy
e-mail: domenico.barbuti@opbg.net; laura.tanturri@opbg.net; marco.cirillo@opbg.net

V. Miele, M. Trinci (eds.), *Imaging Trauma and Polytrauma in Pediatric Patients*,
DOI 10.1007/978-3-319-08524-1_7

consequences. Carty and Pierce [8] showed that among 435 cases of abuse, of 55 initially missed by imaging, 6 (12 %) died and 10 (20 %) survived with a handicap. So in case of suspected abuse, a careful interpretation of skeletal surveys by radiologists with experience in pediatric imaging is mandatory.

7.1 Skeletal Injuries

Skeletal injuries are the most common injuries in NAI; every type and location of fracture has been found in abused children. Fractures are documented in near 50 % of physically abused children and, when present, generally suggest the correct diagnosis. In one large series of 429 abuse-related fractures, 76 % were in the long bones, 8 % in the skull, and 8 % in the rib cage [9]. In Leventhal's study [10], in hospitalized infants with fractures, the proportions of cases attributable to abuse decreased with increasing age.

Particularly, the proportion of fractures attributable to abuse in children <12 months of age was 24.9 %, decreasing to 2.9 % in children from 24 to 35 months of age. In children <12 months, >50 % of the fractures of the ribs, radius/ulna, and tibia/fibula were attributable to abuse, while in this age group, only 30.5 % of femur, 28.1 % of clavicle, and 17.1 % of skull fractures were categorized as abuse.

Children younger than 18 months have immature skeleton and a violent shaking may cause metaphyseal and rib fractures that are highly specific for abuse and are rarely found in older children with abuse-related injury. First described by Caffey [4], metaphyseal fracture is virtually pathognomonic of abuse. Kleinman et al. [7] called this injury "classic metaphyseal lesions" that are a series of microfractures across the metaphysis parallel to the physis, due to shearing injury across the bone end. This type of fractures is seen almost exclusively in children younger than 2 years of age who are small enough to be shaken and are still unable to protect their extremities. Microfractures extend across the metaphysis and may completely or partially cross it; the radiologic appearance is a lucent area within the subphyseal metaphysis, extending across the metaphysis, perpendicular to the long axis of bone. The typical X-ray image is a triangular fragment that if viewed in profile is called "corner fracture" (Fig. 7.1a, b), while if viewed in an oblique angle, the thick rim may be visible as a bowed line termed "bucket-handle fracture" (Fig. 7.1c, d). Although the metaphyseal lesions cause poor clinical findings that are never the main cause of hospitalization and can hardly be suspected by those who take care of the child, these fractures may be dated with precision [1, 7].

7.1.1 Rib Fractures

Rib fractures occur in older children in case of motor vehicle accidents, while in infants without metabolic bone disease, they are extremely rare, thus being highly suggestive of NAI (Fig. 7.2). Fractures of the first rib require even

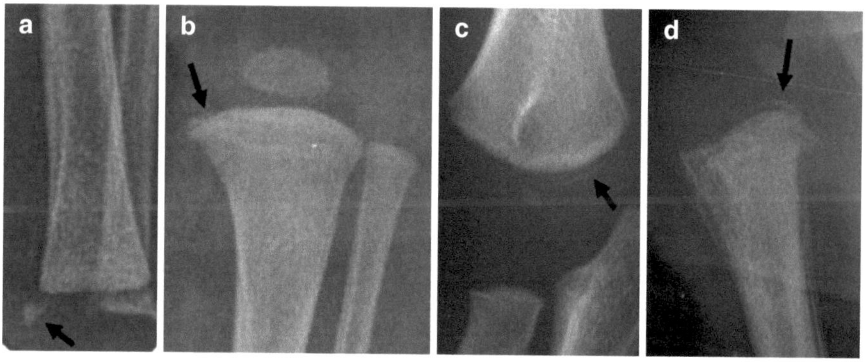

Fig. 7.1 Corner lesion (*arrows* in **a** and **b**) and bucket-handle lesion (*arrows* in **c** and **d**)

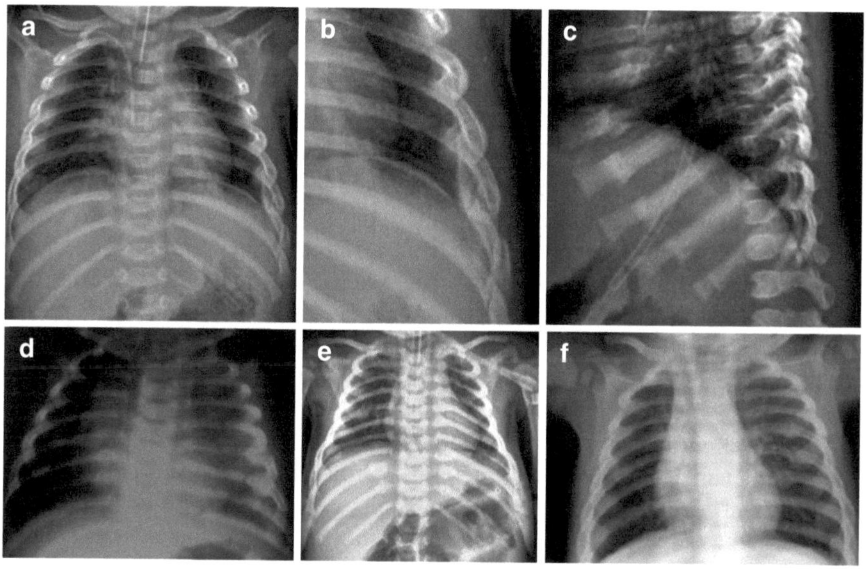

Fig. 7.2 Multiple rib fractures in different stages of evolution (**a–c** same patient; **d–f** other patients)

greater force than other rib fractures and strongly suggest abuse [11]. Barsness et al. [12] examining 62 rib fractures in children found that in the 82 % of cases, the lesions were due to abuse even reaching 95 % in children less than 3 years of age. Due to the plasticity of the young children's skeleton, the rib cage can more easily deform rather than break. Rib fractures in infants are strongly correlated with abuse with a specific mechanism: adult hands pressing the infant chest generates squeezing force on the immature skeleton that may result in fractures of the anterior, lateral, and posterior aspects of the rib [13]. Sometimes, generally in large babies (>3,300 g) with difficult deliveries, rib fracture may be produced by a birth trauma. Posterior rib fracture is highly specific for NAI

Table 7.1 Specificity of radiological findings in child abuse

High specificity	Moderate specificity	Common findings with low specificity
"Classical" metaphyseal lesions	Multiple fractures, especially bilateral	Clavicular fractures
Posterior rib fractures	Several fractures in different healing stage	Diaphyseal fractures of long bones
Scapular fractures	Epiphyseal separations	Linear skull fractures
Spinous process fractures	Vertebral body fractures and subluxations	Subperiosteal new bone formation
Sternal fractures	Digital fractures	
	Complex skull fractures	

given that posteriorly the ribs are attached relatively tightly to the vertebral bodies and transverse processes. Since the forces are distributed in an area similar to the size of adult's hands, fractures are typically seen in similar locations in multiple adjacent ribs and are often bilateral. Fracture healing occurs rapidly and may be divided into four stages: inflammation, soft callus, hard callus, and remodeling. Acute rib fractures appear as complete or incomplete linear lucent areas across the rib; however, if the fracture is incomplete or complete but nondisplaced or in an area with many overlapping structures, it may be hard to visualize, especially at the costovertebral joint. With healing, more fractures become apparent, as subperiosteal new bone and callus become evident. Thus, follow-up radiography performed 2 weeks after the injury increases the detection of rib fractures. Oblique chest radiography and bone scintigraphy are helpful to increase the detection of fractures. It has been shown that bone isotopic scan demonstrates radiographically occult rib fractures in 10 % of abused children [14]. Computed tomography (CT) performed in presence of polytrauma can easily depict rib fractures. Cardiopulmonary resuscitation may result in rib fractures more commonly in adults generally involving the anterior ribs, while posterior rib fracture does not result from such maneuvers. The rib fractures located on the middle axillary line have no distinctive characteristics from those determined by resuscitation. Spevak et al. [15] reported 0 % of rib fractures on autopsy in 91 infants who died after cardiac resuscitation, and Sewell reported no rib fracture after prolonged cardiac massage in a case of osteogenesis imperfecta type II [16]. Specificities of X-ray findings for infant abuse are listed in Table 7.1.

7.1.2 Other Fractures

Any type of fracture has been described in NAI. Particular attention should be given to the age and development of the child as well as to the injury and its mechanism. The given history for the injury is extremely important since it reveals the degree of

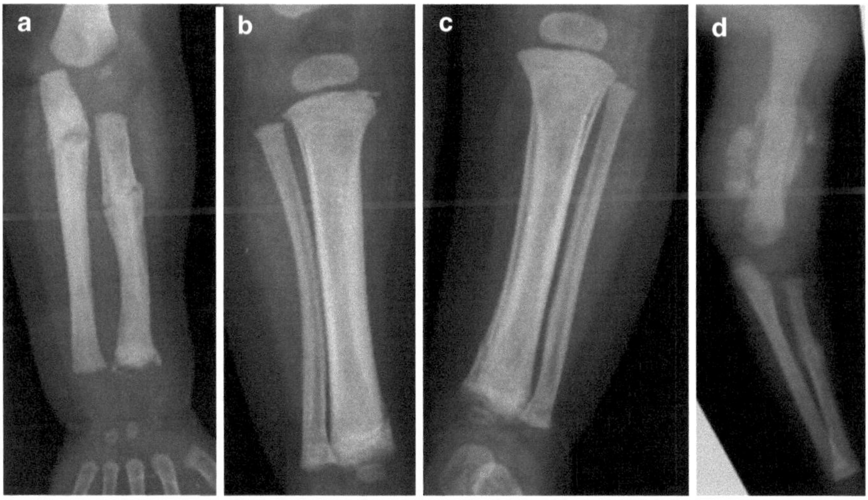

Fig. 7.3 Multiple fractures of long bones in different stages of healing (**a–c** on the same patient: radioulnar and tibioperoneal fractures; (**d**) another patient with humeral and radial fracture in different stages of healing)

force of the injury. Physeal fractures are rare under 3 years old. Type I Salter-Harris fractures in infants are not simply identified in the acute phase since the epiphysis is not ossified; thus, US can help in the correct diagnosis. Diaphyseal fractures of long bones are a common finding in children with a low specificity for abuse; this type of fractures generally occur as a result of accidental trauma in older children, while they are suspected for abuse in non-walking infants; "those who don't cruise, don't bruise" [17]. Multiple diaphyseal fractures in different stages of healing are shown in Fig. 7.3. Pelvic fractures in young children generally are due to motor vehicle accidents and, however, have been reported in NAI [18]. The domestic accidents as a fall from a high chair, a changing table, a sofa, a baby crib, or a bed are common and rarely lead to fractures or other serious injuries. A fall down the stairs is often used as an explanation for an inflicted injury, but epidemiologic studies of stairway falls demonstrate a limited injury pattern. In walking children, spiral fracture of the tibia called "toddler fracture" (Fig. 7.4) is common without a clear precedent trauma; it is not suspected of abuse, although it is often diagnosed already in the initial phase of healing because the child refuses to walk. Any vertebral fracture in children without a good explanation is suspected for NAI.

7.1.3 Fracture Healing in Children

Infants heal more quickly than older children and adults do. Dating the age of fractures in suspected abused children is very important, especially in the presence of more than one fracture and when the given history is suspect. The subperiosteal

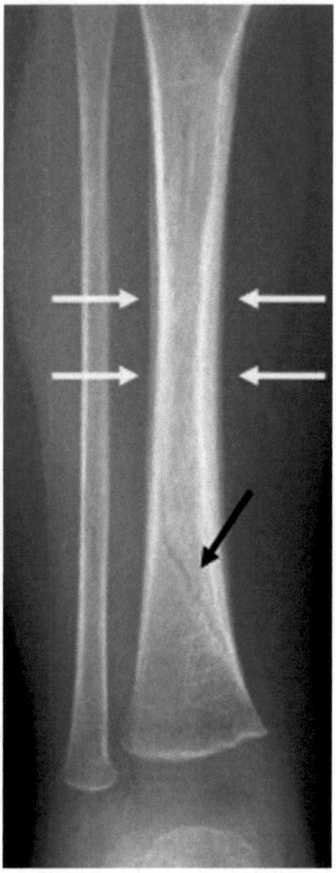

Fig. 7.4 Toddler fracture: oblique metaphyseal fracture (*black arrow*) diagnosed during healing phase with slight periosteal reaction (*white arrows*). This fracture is not suspected for NAI

new bone (soft callus) is visible within 10 days after the injury. Calcified, and so visible, callus is observed in all fractures after 2–4 weeks (Fig. 7.5). Incomplete bridging of the fracture line is noted as early as 3 weeks after injury, and complete bridging with disappearance of fracture lucency is evident in almost half of the fractures at 10 weeks. Metaphyseal fractures can be dated with a good approximation: at a short distance from trauma, it is possible to detect marginal fragments of the physis and laminar gaps of the metaphyseal cortex; then, a progressive cortico-periosteal reaction occurs followed by the complete fusion of the fracture fragments to meta-diaphyseal region. Repeated and not treated subperiosteal hemorrhages determine after a few weeks the formation of thick periosteal sleeve and subsequently the cupping deformation of the metaphyses producing permanent alterations of the limbs such as bowing and dysmetria. Radiologists should be able to distinguish recent from old fractures, to determine if a fracture (excluding skull fractures) is in phase of healing as well as to recognize whether the fractures are of similar or different age in presence of multiple fractures.

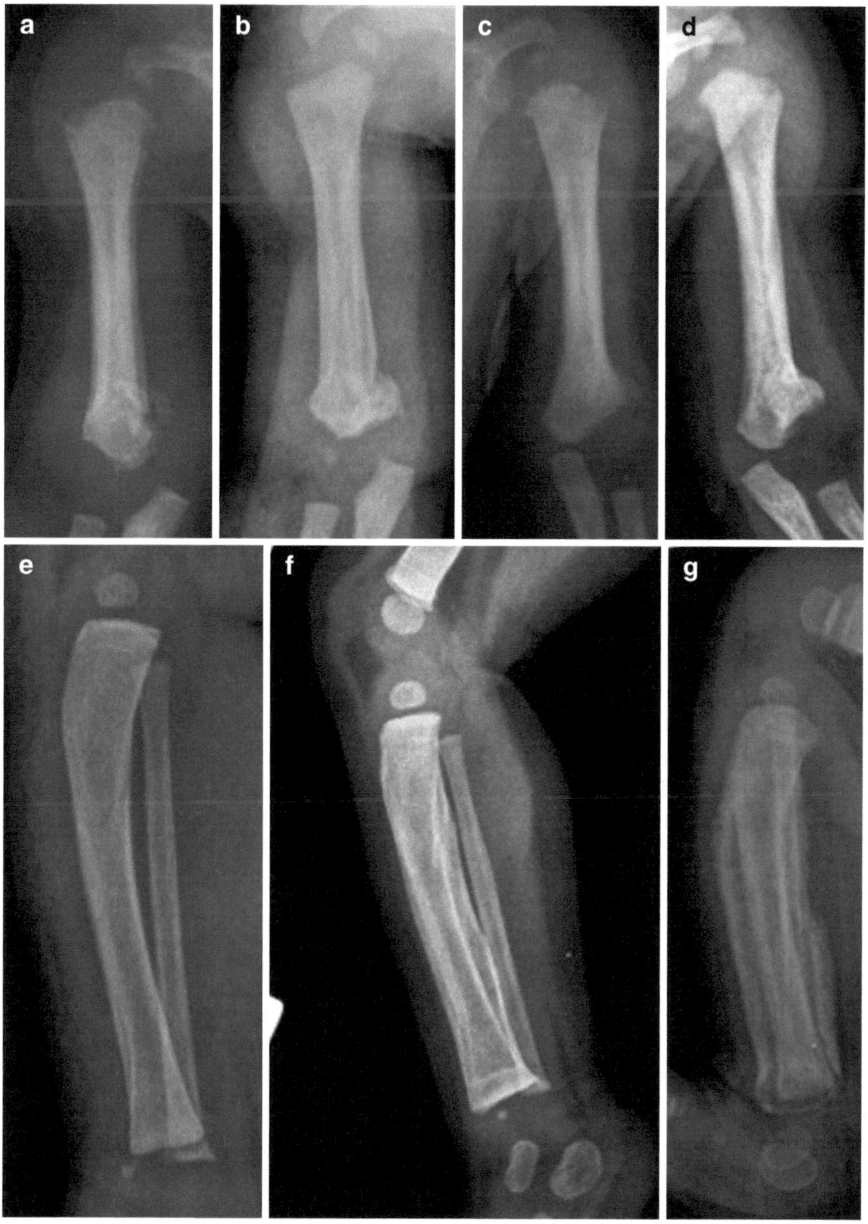

Fig. 7.5 Repair process: (**a**) *right humerus*: partial detachment associated with reparative periosteal apposition. (**b**) After 2 weeks complete fusion of the fracture fragment (**c**) *left humerus*: corner lesion (**c**) and complete repair after 2 weeks (**d**); (**e**) distal tibial corner fracture; (**f**) large periosteal apposition after 10 days and complete healing after 38 days (**g**)

7.2 X-Ray of the Skeleton

X-ray of the skeleton is the first study in suspected NAI if the baby is in a stable condition. In order to make a correct diagnosis, X-rays need to be technically well done. Skeletal radiograph allows:

- To detect a hidden damage to the bone
- To get additional information about a clinically suspected NAI
- To date the injury
- To discover any disorder of the musculoskeletal system that can predispose to a fracture

The X-ray study must be carried out in a technically correct way and must be of high diagnostic quality. The right timing of the X-ray allows the early identification of a NAI and an immediate alert of the security team in order to promptly support the child. In fact, a delay in the examination might help parents to provide an alibi as declaring that the trauma occurred during hospitalization. When the child refers to the Department of Diagnostic Imaging, the radiological staff must be in contact with the staff that takes care of the child so that the X-ray is performed in the most appropriate time, and after the examination the child can go back to the clinical reference for ongoing care, thus suggesting the need of a multidisciplinary assessment. The X-ray must be made in accordance with the principles of accuracy and radiological high quality, which include highly technical factors, patient positioning, correct exposure factors for age and weight, and appropriate protections. In all radiographs, the name of the patient, a side marker studied, the date, and the time of the test must be clearly and correctly visible. The radiologist may request additional views if necessary. It is important that each anatomical area is examined with a separate exposure in order to optimize image quality. In particular, the whole skeleton ("babygram") should not be performed on a single X-ray. Soft tissues as well as bone must be studied, since soft tissue swelling can be an indirect sign of fracture.

The radiographic views that should be performed in all cases of suspected NAI are shown in Table 7.2. X-rays are of extreme importance during the follow-up too, in order to confirm or exclude the diagnosis of NAI. The X-ray follow-up substantially increases the discovery of rib and metaphyseal fractures. In case of strong suspicion of NAI, it is necessary to perform a complete X-ray of the skeleton (except the skull) for the detection of occult fractures not seen on the first X-ray examination. In case of equivocal findings, in some areas at the first examination, it is necessary to repeat screenings of these anatomical areas to demonstrate radiographic signs suggestive of bone healing. The timing of the follow-up is crucial for dating the fractures. Radiographic examination should be repeated approximately 2 weeks after the first examination (from 11 to 14 days), even if this behavior has potential drawbacks: delay in diagnosis in some cases, inability to properly handle the child and his family as a result of delay, difficulty in deciding the place in which the child will stay in the interval between the first and the second examination, and possibility that the child will miss the X-ray follow-up. In our hospital, we use a system of flat

Table 7.2 The skeletal survey in suspected infant abuse

Anteroposterior chest including clavicles
Lateral chest
Anteroposterior humeri
Anteroposterior forearms
Posteroanterior hands
Anteroposterior pelvis
Lateral lumbar spine
Anteroposterior femora
Anteroposterior tibiae
Anteroposterior feet
Anteroposterior skull
Lateral skull

Note: All positive sites should be viewed in at least two projections. The expert radiologist will decide to perform further radiographic views if necessary

panel detectors ("flat panel detectors," FPD), which result in a higher image quality and in a substantial X-ray exposure reduction. In newborns, the kV range used for radiographic examination of all the skeletal segments ranges from 55 to 70. The focus-film distance is ~100 cm. Both joints should be included in the examinations of the long bones. Chest X-ray should be performed using the bone technique. The radiology report should provide a concise description of all the areas where a fracture is present or suspected. It is very important to collect precise informations about the event. The inconsistent responses should not be contradicted. The radiologist's goal in the suspected NAI is to identify injury by imaging (in agreement with ALARA – *As Low As Reasonably Achievable*), to check the congruence between history and lesions diagnosed, to determine whether the etiology of the lesions is virtually non-accidental, to discover the age of injury, and, in doubt of abuse, to cooperate with physicians, coroner, magistrate, etc. [19].

7.2.1 Radioisotopic Bone Scanning

Scintigraphy is extremely sensitive in the identification of fractures and in some cases is able to demonstrate traumatic lesions invisible or hardly detectable at the first X-ray of the skeleton. Considered together, radiography and skeletal scintigraphy identify a greater number of traumatic injuries. CT has the same role in NAI and in accidental bone trauma. It is able to define the extent and severity of complex fractures and/or fractures unrecognized by X-ray and in particular vertebral, sternal, scapular, pelvic, and complex joint fractures. MRI has a prominent role in the evaluation of soft tissue trauma, occurring alone or in association with skeletal trauma. Recently some authors emphasized the role of whole-body MRI with STIR sequences and Fluorine-18 NaF PET imaging for the study of skeletal lesions instead of skeletal survey [20, 21].

7.2.2 Postmortem Radiography

Children who die from a sudden and unexpected or unexplained death generally undergo autopsy to determine the cause of death. X-rays is needed to complete the autopsy and in doubt of abuse should be performed in a small field of view in order to highlight rib fractures and typical metaphyseal lesions that can suggest the diagnosis of NAI. Therefore, a postmortem radiographic skeletal survey must be done in all children who die under suspicious circumstances in the hospital before transporting to the coroner's office.

7.3 Visceral Lesions

Thoraco-abdominal visceral lesions from NAI are not common, representing 2–4 % of injuries. This type of lesions are described in all ages but are most common in children less than 3 years, with a high mortality rate (around 45–53 %) especially due to diagnostic and therapeutic delay [22]. Lesions of the hollow viscera are rarely found in accidental trauma in which single lesions of solid organs are most frequent; thus, they are highly suggestive of abuse. The injury can be caused by collision of solid organs against the spine, by compression of the hollow viscera against the column, by acceleration or deceleration of mobile structures, and rarely from blowout. Young children are more vulnerable because the ribs are more subtle, abdominal organs are more prominent, the abdominal walls are thinner, the muscles and skeletal structures are weaker compared to adult, and there is little protective fatty tissue around the pancreas, kidneys, and bowel loops. Most injuries occur in the duodenum (Fig. 7.6a, b) (with a prevalence of parietal hematoma due to the rich vascularization) and in proximal jejunum (with a prevalence of perforation due to the relatively fixed position) [23]. In stable patients, in case of suspect of visceral lesions, contrast-enhanced CT is the first investigation. It allows good evaluation of the lesion, shows the presence of free air or endo-abdominal fluid, and is the method of choice to detect lesions of the small bowel and mesentery. For an accurate diagnosis, it is important to get the correct timing of the contrast bolus. The examination should be performed without oral contrast medium, which could increase the risk of aspiration, especially if a child is sedated or immobilized. Protocols should be used with doses as low as possible (ALARA) in relation to the weight of the child, for example, not more than 80 KV in neonates and infants, directly after infusion of contrast medium. US has low sensitivity for lesions of solid organs and viscera and does not evaluate the bones and lungs; thus, it can be useful only in minor trauma and during follow-up of parenchymal lesions. In the chest pulmonary contusions, pleural effusion, cardiac laceration, esophageal rupture, aortic dissection, aortic pseudoaneurysm by direct trauma, and lethal "commotio cordis" are described [24]. In the abdomen, rarely can occur a gastric rupture with rapid onset of painful symptoms that can lead, especially if the diagnosis is delayed, to sepsis, shock, and death. Intramural hematoma in young children generally indicates abuse since it can be

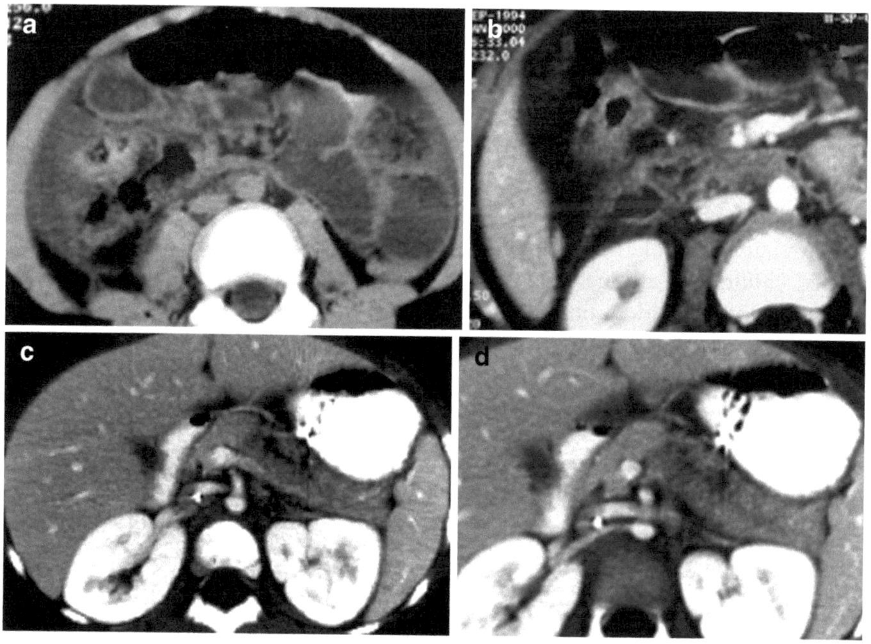

Fig. 7.6 Duodenal perforation (**a**, **b**) with fluid effusion. Pancreas laceration (**c**, **d**)

spontaneous only in case of purpura or coagulation disorders. It is manifested by partial or complete obstruction but often the symptoms appear late. Pancreas lesions are due to direct trauma to the upper abdomen. A complete pancreatic transection can occur (Fig. 7.6c, d) with a possible subsequent development of pseudocyst. Pancreatic lesions can evolve in early or late pancreatitis; in fact, pancreatitis in young children without a familiar history is suspected of abuse [25]. Visceral injuries are often associated to pancreatic lesions. Liver lesions are not frequent nor characteristics of NAI. The bleeding can be contained by the liver capsule or it can reach the peritoneal cavity. Most liver lesions are treated conservatively. Splenic and urinary tract lesions are not common in abuse and may be associated with other alterations. A scrotal hematoma can be caused by direct trauma or by extravasation of blood from the abdomen. There may be lesions of the penis. Vascular lesions are rare in children. Intra-abdominal vessels lesions are rare and may be associated with other lesions of the liver or the spleen.

7.4 Non-accidental Head Injuries (NAHI)

A non-accidental head injury occurs in about 12 % of abused children and in children under 2 years of age, representing 80 % of deaths from head trauma. In children aged less than 1 year, 95 % of all serious intracranial injuries and 64 % of all head injuries were the result of child abuse [26]. The prognosis of head trauma from abuse is significantly worse than that from an accidental head injury. NAHI in infants is associated with 12.5–40 % mortality rate [27]. Disabilities and mental retardation are common sequelae of abuse in children who survive.

7.4.1 Skull Fractures

Skull fractures are relatively common in both accidental and caused injuries. In the abused children in all age groups, skull fractures account for about 8–13 % of fractures, but in children under 2 years of age, the percentage rises to 29–33 %. A fracture of the skull has been discovered in up to 41 % of pediatric homicide [28]. Skull fractures result from trauma with a contact, while a child skull deformation causes injury to the brain and the meninges without fractures. Wider and more soft is the contact surface, where less likely a fracture occurs. An area of close contact with sufficient speed will result in a depressed fracture of the skull. The infant skull is relatively plastic and deformable; thus, it is more resistant to fracture, so in many studies, skull fractures occur in only 1–3 % of children falling from a height of 6 ft or less [29]. Surprisingly in domestic trauma although skull fractures are frequent, a significant brain damage (with the exception of epidural hematoma) is rare; 95 % of skull fractures with serious injuries in hospitalized children less than 2 years of age are from abuse [1]. Fractures of the skull cannot be dated with precision, and a radiolucent line may be visible on X-ray until 6/12 months after the trauma; multiple fractures, fractures that cross suture, bilateral fractures, and fractures with diastasis greater than 3 mm are more likely associated with abuse. According to some authors [30], the skull X-ray is preferable to CT because fracture lines that have parallel or nearly parallel orientation of the section may not be visible on CT. The radiographic examination of the skull in the anteroposterior and lateral views is part of the skeletal survey, with additional views (Towne, the opposite side L-L, Waters), if necessary. The fractures appear as radiolucent images with sharp edges linear or branched. A diastasis of 3 mm or more can occur (Fig. 7.7). Scintigraphy is not recommended since it is poorly sensitive for skull fractures. In case of polytrauma, the patient directly undergoes a CT examination.

7.4.2 Extra-axial Hemorrhage

Subdural hemorrhage (SDH) and subarachnoid hemorrhage (SAH) are common injuries in trauma from abuse, while the epidural hematoma is much more often accidental. In 287 children aged between 1 week and 6.5 years with head injuries, SDH was found in 46 % and SAH in 31 % of abused children (compared with 10 and 8 %, respectively, in children with accidental head trauma) [31]. A subdural interhemispheric hematoma has the highest specificity for abuse of any intracranial lesion, although it can also be caused by motor vehicle accidents. The mechanism is a "back and forth" movement with laceration of the midline veins. Subdural hematoma appears

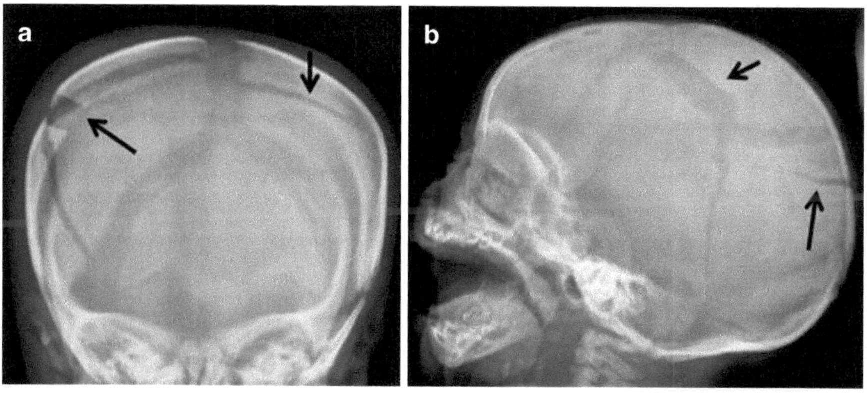

Fig. 7.7 Skull fracture with diastasis of the fragments (*arrows*) in A-P (**a**) and L-L (**b**) view

as an interhemispheric (parafalcine) collection. SDH classically appears on CT as an area of high attenuation when the bleeding is acute, while it becomes isodense compared to the brain and, finally, hypodense after days or weeks [32]. In acute SDH, active bleeding can appear as a not uniform hyperdensity which can be misdiagnosed as a subacute SDH or multiple SDHs [33]. Recently US with Doppler has been used to study the extra-axial cerebrospinal fluid (CSF) spaces in infant brain [34]. US is very useful in differentiating diffuse enlargement of the subarachnoid spaces (benign external hydrocephalus of childhood) from SDH, which unlikely can be identified on CT. In US the subarachnoid space is characterized by an anechoic fluid crossed by multiple vessels parallel to the cortex (cortical veins), and the lack of such vessels might suggest the presence of meningitis or SDH. Limits of US are poor visualization of the posterior fossa and areas far from anterior fontanelle and the inability to distinguish the nature of abnormal fluid collections such as SDH and meningitis [34]. US is very useful in the follow-up of anomalies previously documented by CT or MR.

7.4.3 Brain Parenchymal Lesions

The damage of the brain parenchyma occurs at the junction between white and gray matter; the different densities of the brain tissue make it particularly susceptible to shear forces (axonal damage). Axonal damage is due to traumatic axonal stretching (rarely disconnection) secondary to sudden acceleration/deceleration associated with rotational/angular forces. Such injuries can be microscopic or macroscopic and focal (Fig. 7.8a–e) or diffuse and are typical of infants aged less than 5 months [35]. It has been demonstrated [36] that the diffuse axonal injury (DAI), once considered the most important component of NAHI, is less frequent than diffuse cerebral edema and affects 40 % of children with NAHI. The symptom of DAI is impaired consciousness without lucid intervals. The most affected locations are the gray-white junction, the corpus callosum, the brain stem, and the basal ganglia.

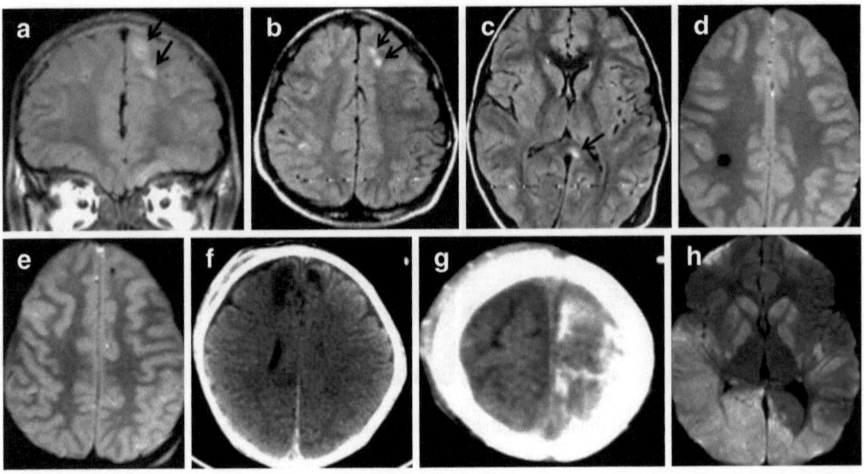

Fig. 7.8 (**a–e**) focal axonal injury in the frontal lobe (*arrows* in **a** and **b**) and in the splenium of the corpus callosum (*arrow* in **c**); (**d–e**) in T2* sequences two small areas of signal void due to hemosiderin; (**f–g**) CT scans several bleedings differently aged in another child; (**h**) cerebral edema in FLAIR sequence (Courtesy of Bruno Bernardi, MD Chief of Neuroradiology OPBG, Rome)

7.4.4 Cerebral Contusion

Cerebral contusion is a focal hemorrhage (Fig. 7.8f, g) within the brain parenchyma which derives from direct contact forces. These lesions are very rare in infants and are usually small and therefore difficult to detect on CT. Cerebral contusions generally involve the cortex of the frontal and temporal lobes and the parafalcine areas. MR is more accurate in detecting such lesions; particularly, gradient echo sequences are extremely useful in order to detect small amounts of hemoglobin. The areas of brain contusion may develop into focal areas of encephalomalacia with cystic cavities.

7.4.5 Cerebral Edema

Focal or diffuse cerebral edema (Fig. 7.8h) is a common feature of NAHI. It can be the expression of the primary lesion or the consequence of hypoxia by strangulation, suffocation, or prolonged apnea. On CT, edema appears as a focal or diffuse hypodensity associated with loss of distinction between gray and white matter, causing a mass effect if extended. On MRI, cortical edema appears as hyperintensity on T2-weighted images. In newborn/small infants, the white matter, still not myelinated, has a high water content; thus, edema of the white matter may be not easily detected. In these patients, diffusion-weighted imaging (DWI) is a valuable diagnostic tool; particularly it can detect early cytotoxic edema with areas of restriction of the diffusion of water appearing bright; moreover DWI can demonstrate early ischemic lesions and generally NAHI are more extensive on DWI compared with other MRI sequences. The clinical outcome of intracranial trauma from abuse is generally worse than that from road accidents [37]. A cervical lesion is rarely found in abused patients [38]. Studies of pathological anatomy have supported the hypothesis that the brain injury is actually a pontine, medullary, cervical, and basal nuclei hypoxic-ischemic lesion caused by cardiorespiratory changes from mechanical injury [39]. According to this theory, flexion and hyperextension of the neck during the shaking, especially in younger children in which the weight of the head is greater in percentage compared to the trunk and the infants are not able to support the head well, may cause acute or chronic injury to the brain. However, this theory does not explain SDH and retinal hemorrhages. Therefore, since the injury mechanisms are not yet completely clear and there is no agreement in the literature on them, the term "shaken baby" has been replaced by "non-accidental head injuries" (NAHI) [40].

7.5 Role of CT and MRI in Suspected NAHI

CT is highly sensitive and specific in the assessment of acute intracranial hemorrhage and parenchymal hypodense lesions as in cerebral edema, ischemia, and infarction. The CT scans must be acquired from the skull base to the vertex, with a thickness equal or lower than 5 mm. In case of MDCT, a cranial volume is taken from the vertex to the second cervical vertebra and reconstructed in the axial coronal and sagittal and 3D planes at 2–3 mm slices. The images must be displayed with a window suitable for the study of soft tissues and bone and with an intermediate window in the presence of very small extra-axial hematomas. MRI is more accurate in the assessment of parenchymal changes in the acute phase and allows a better mapping in intracranial subacute and chronic hemorrhage. MRI findings in the course of hemorrhage vary according to time due to the metabolism of hemoglobin. In children under 2–3 months of age, a surface coil for the knee can be used for the best signal/noise ratio, while in older children the skull coil is generally used. Before 12 months, since myelin is not completely formed and the brain has a high water content, it might be useful to increase the TR on T2-weighted sequences, which determine an increase of the contrast between white and gray matter. The images on DWI should be obtained routinely for an earlier diagnosis of brain lesions and for the assessment of the ischemic lesions. The combined use of CT and MRI allows a more accurate detection, localization, and characterization of intracranial trauma and a better monitoring of brain injury. The late effects of head trauma are better evaluated with MRI and include large chronic subdural hematoma/CSF collection, hydrocephalus, and leptomeningeal cyst in "growing fractures."

The diagnostic algorithm in suspected NAHI is shown in Table 7.3.

Table 7.3 Flowchart of diagnostic tests in suspected NAHI

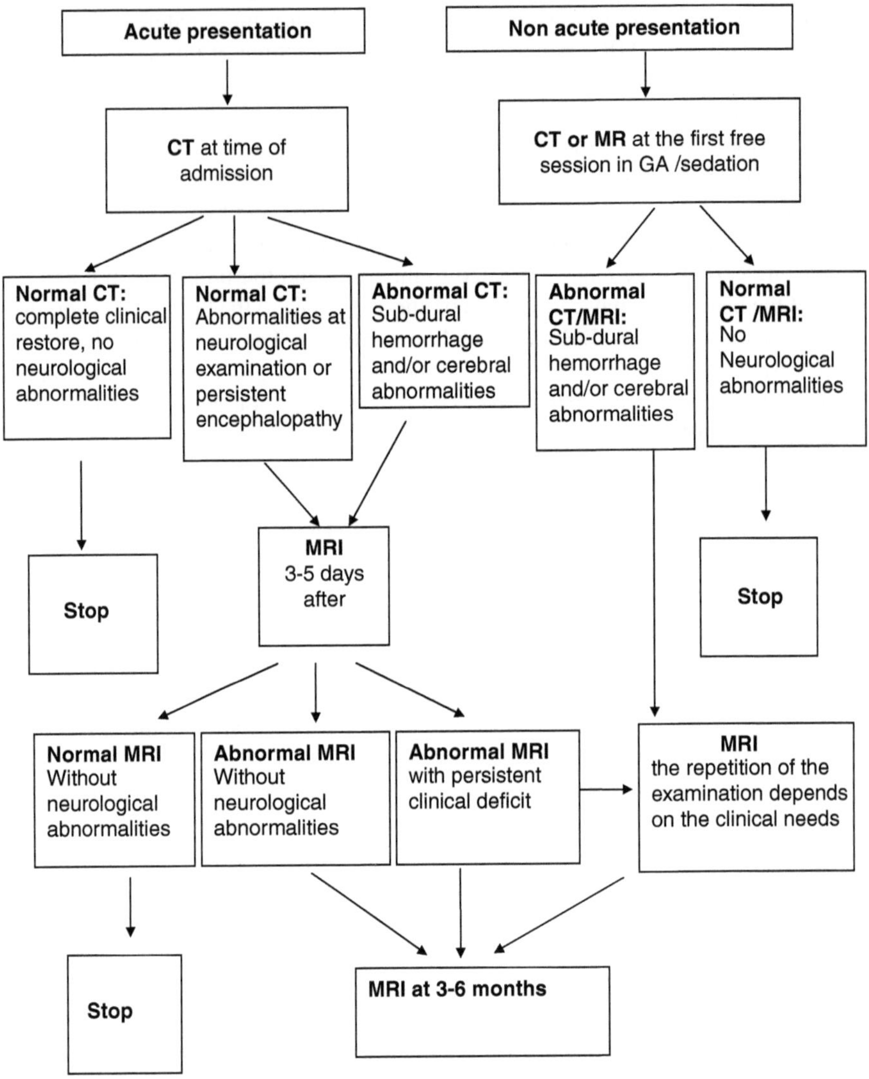

7.6 Differential Diagnosis of NAI

1. Birth injury. It is seen more frequently in newborn with a difficult delivery and in children of high weight. More affected bones are the clavicle (usually at the middle third, while in NAI at the lateral end, (Fig. 7.9a, b)), humerus, and femur. Even if rare, epiphyseal separations (on elbow, hip, humerus) and rib fractures can be also determined. The callus is typically visible on X-ray after a week; thus, a fracture without reparative phenomena in infants aged 7–10 days is suspected for NAI.

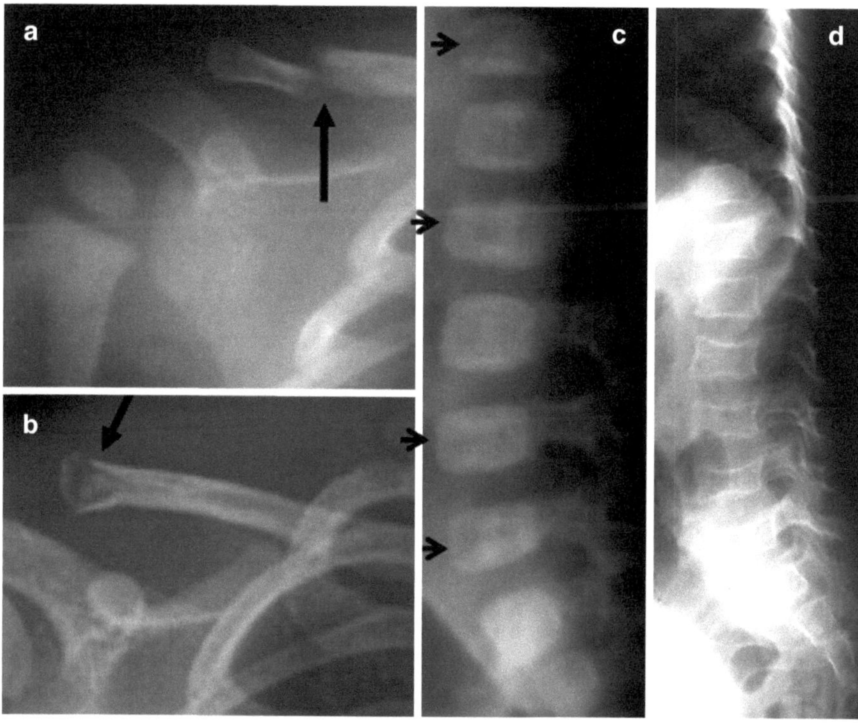

Fig. 7.9 Differential diagnosis of NAI: birth fracture of the clavicle (*arrow* in **a**), third middle; fracture of the clavicle from NAI, third lateral (*arrow* in **b**). A fracture in infants 7–10 days old without repair phenomena is NOT a birth fracture but is suspected for NAI! Multiple partial vertebral collapses in NAI (*arrows* in **c**) and in osteogenesis imperfecta (**d**): osteoporosis and multiple "sprocket" vertebrae

2. Osteogenesis imperfecta and other congenital bone dysplasias. Osteogenesis imperfecta is a genetic disease classified into 7 types. It is characterized by multiple rib, vertebral, and long bones fractures in different developmental stage. However, the serious and diffuse reduction in the tone of calcium, the presence of multiple Wormian bones in the skull, the presence of blue sclera (except type V), the bowing bones in the "thin bones" forms, or the deformity in the "thick bones" forms (type II) helps in the diagnosis (Fig. 7.9c, d). In metaphyseal chondrodysplasia Schmid type, the metaphyseal abnormalities resemble the previously described "corner lesions." Menkes disease with abnormal hair, metaphyseal spurs, and massive subdural hematoma can mimic NAI too [41].
3. Infantile cortical hyperostosis (De Tony-Caffey-Silverman disease). It usually affects infants in the first 2 months of life. Clinical signs are fever, malaise, and painful swelling of the affected limbs. Generally acute symptoms resolve spontaneously in a few months. It is characterized by periosteal apposition. The scapula and the mandible.
4. Osteopathy of prematurity. The premature neonate often suffers from osteoporosis, rickets, and metaphyseal abnormalities, and in the most serious forms,

pathological fractures and subperiosteal hematoma can be observed too. The disease is due to mineral deficiencies and to insufficient uptake of calcium and vitamin D from parenteral nutrition. The history of prematurity, severe osteoporosis, and laboratory tests can suggest the correct diagnosis.

5. Rickets. In the various forms of rickets, flare "cupped" metaphyses with fraying and bowing of the lower limbs, long bones are often affected by pathological fractures. The enlargement of the physis and the typical radiological signs usually allow the correct diagnosis.
6. Congenital lues. The symptoms of *Treponema pallidum* infection, which is a reemerging problem related to immigration, appear at birth or, more often, few weeks after birth with skeletal and abdominal involvement and pseudoparalysis of Parrot. The metaphyses of long bones can be affected. Particularly dystrophic striae, fragmentation and erosion and the typical Wimberger sign, symmetrical erosion of the metaphysis of proximal tibia, and hyperostosis of the diaphyses can be observed. All this signs can mimic NAI but laboratory tests can easily clarify the diagnosis.
7. Scurvy. Scurvy is a rare disease due to vitamin C deficiency which can occur in infants [42]. The principal signs of the disease are bruising and bleeding gums, pain, and functional impotence and fragmentation of the metaphysis at skeletal survey. An experienced radiologist can easily make the correct diagnosis, later confirmed by low dose of ascorbic acid.
8. Temporary brittle bone disease [43]. It is characterized by multiple fractures during the first year of age. During follow-up, any type of fracture can be observed. It generally affects premature neonates, especially twins. Common features are apnea, colic, family history of joint laxity, and copper malabsorption. The disease is controversial and not universally accepted.

7.7 Conclusions

NAI is an important cause of death and morbidity, especially in young children. Some patterns of lesions are highly suggestive of non-accidental trauma, and therefore, it is essential to recognize the typical radiological signs. NAI should always be considered among the diagnostic hypotheses in case of trauma with multiple fractures in different stages of healing in children younger than 2 years and/or fractures in atypical locations and with uncommon features, such as metaphyseal lesions, posterior rib fractures, and fractures of sternum or scapula especially if associated with intracranial hemorrhage, and finally in every case of injury with unclear explanations. If the final diagnosis of NAI has been established, the study should not be limited to the musculoskeletal system since injuries to other organs can occur and can lead to death if undetected. In fact, about 2–4 % of children hospitalized for trauma from abuse present abdominal injuries, with a high mortality rate, being the second most common cause of death in fatal abuse. The NAHI represents only 12 % of the physical injuries from abuse but is the leading cause of death in the abused children under 2 years of life and the most common cause of traumatic death in infancy. The clinical manifestations are often not clear and may be misdiagnosed.

A simple "alphabet" could be proposed for NAI:

A. *Anamnesis*: Are the informations consistent and not changed? Explain the lesions.
B. *Biomechanics*: Are the characteristics of fractures consistent with the biomechanics produced by the described trauma?
C. *Chronology*: Are signs, symptoms, and behaviors congruent with fractures? Are the lesions consistent with the mental and physical development of the patient? Was the child care delayed?
D. *Dermatology*: Are skin lesions (contusions, abrasions, bruises, burns, etc.) compatible with the data collected in anamnesis and with the skeletal lesions? Are the skin lesions suspected for a not accidental etiology?

Red flags of NAI are:

Age: <18 months, 80 % of cases.
Anamnesis: vague and contradictory. Reported behavior of the child does not fit with patient's age and psychomotor ability.
Time: delay in the hospital admission.
Skin lesions: unexplained lesions, not compatible with the described trauma.
Fractures: must be compatible with the biomechanics of the trauma. Fractures of high specificity are metaphyseal lesions, posterior rib fractures, fractures of the sternum and the scapula, and fractures of fingers and toes in children who do not walk. Fractures not otherwise explained (e.g., car accident) are highly suggestive of NAI. Several fractures at different stages of healing are expression of multiple repeated trauma.

References

1. Lonergan GJ, Baker AM, Morey MK et al (2003) Child abuse: radiologic-pathologic correlation. Radiographics 23:811–845
2. Tardieu A (1860) Etude medico-legale sur les services et mauvais traitments exerces sur des infants. Ann Hyg Publ Med Leg 13:361–398
3. Caffey J (1946) Multiple fractures in the long bones of infants suffering from chronic subdural hematoma. Am J Roentgenol Radium Ther Nucl Med 56:163–173
4. Caffey J (1957) Some traumatic lesions in growing bones other than fractures and dislocations: clinical and radiological features. Br J Radiol 30:225–238
5. Kempe CH, Silverman FN, Steele BF et al (1962) The battered-child syndrome. JAMA 181:105–112
6. Guthkelch AN (1971) Infantile subdural haematoma and its relationship to whiplash injuries. Br Med J 2:430–431
7. Kleinman PK, Marks SC, Blackbourne B (1986) The metaphyseal lesion in abused infants: a radiologic-histopathologic study. AJR Am J Roentgenol 146:895–905

8. Carty H, Pierce A (2002) Non-accidental injury: a retrospective analysis of a large cohort. Eur Radiol 12:2919–2925
9. King J, Diefendorf D, Apthorp J et al (1988) Analysis of 429 fractures in 189 battered children. J Pediatr Orthop 8:585–589
10. Leventhal JM, Martin KD, Asnes AG (2008) Incidence of fractures attributable to abuse in young hospitalized children: results from analysis of a United States database. Pediatrics 122(3):599–604
11. Strouse PJ, Owings CL (1995) Fractures of the first rib in child abuse. Radiology 197:763–765
12. Barsness KA, Cha ES, Bensard DD et al (2003) The positive predictive value of rib fractures as an indicator of nonaccidental trauma in children. J Trauma 54:1107–1110
13. Offiah A, van Rijn RR, Perez-Rossello JM et al (2009) Skeletal imaging of child abuse (non-accidental injury). Pediatr Radiol 39:461–470
14. Sty JR, Starshak RJ (1983) The role of bone scintigraphy in the evaluation of the suspected abused child. Radiology 146:369–375
15. Spevak MR, Kleinman PK, Belanger PL, Primack C, Richmond JM (1994) Cardiopulmonary resuscitation and rib fractures in infants: a postmortem radiologic- pathologic study. JAMA 272:617–618
16. Sewell RD, Steinberg MA (2000) Chest compressions in an infant with osteogenesis imperfecta type II: no new rib fractures. Pediatrics 106(5):E71
17. Sugar NF, Taylor JA, Feldman KW (1999) Bruises in infants and toddlers: those who don't cruise rarely bruise. Puget Sound Pediatric Research Network. Arch Pediatr Adolesc Med 153:399–403
18. Starling SP, Heller RM, Jenny C (2002) Pelvic fractures in infants as a sign of physical abuse. Child Abuse Negl 26:475–480
19. De Filippi C, Santoro B, Pautasso P (2009) Bony lesions from a non-accidental trauma. In: Martino F, De Filippi C, Caudana R (eds) Imaging of pediatric bone and joint trauma. Springer, Milan, pp 187–202
20. Stranzinger E, Kellenberger CJ, Braunschweig S et al (2007) Whole-body STIR MR imaging in suspected child abuse: an alternative to skeletal survey radiography? Eur J Radiol Extra 63:43–47
21. Drubach LA, Sapp MV, Laffin S et al (2008) Fluorine-18 NaF PET imaging of child abuse. Pediatr Radiol 38:776–779
22. Sivit CJ, Taylor GA, Eichelberger MR (1989) Visceral injury in battered children: a changing perspective. Radiology 173:659–661
23. Kunin JR, Korobkin M, Ellis JH et al (1993) Duodenal injuries caused by blunt abdominal trauma: value of CT in differentiating perforation from hematoma. AJR Am J Roentgenol 160:1221–1223
24. Baker AM, Craig BR, Lonergan GJ (2003) Homicidal commotio cordis: the final blow in a battered infant. Child Abuse Negl 27:125–130
25. Swischuk LE (2000) Emergency imaging of the acutely Ill or injured child, 4th edn. Lippincott Williams & Wilkins, Philadelphia
26. Billmire ME, Myers PA (1985) Serious head injury in infants: accident or abuse? Pediatrics 75:340–342
27. Duhaime AC, Alario AJ, Lewander WJ (1992) Head injury in very young children: mechanisms, injury types, and ophthalmologic findings in 100 hospitalized patients younger than 2 years of age. Pediatrics 90:179–185
28. Kleinman PK, Marks SC Jr, Richmond JM et al (1995) Inflicted skeletal injury: a postmortem radiologic-histopathologic study in 31 infants. AJR Am J Roentgenol 165:647–650
29. Lyons TJ, Oates RK (1993) Falling out of bed: a relatively benign occurrence. Pediatrics 92:125–127
30. Saulsbury FT, Alford BA (1982) Intracranial bleeding from child abuse: the value of skull radiographs. Pediatr Radiol 12:175–178

31. Reece RM, Sege R (2000) Childhood head injuries: accidental or inflicted? Arch Pediatr Adolesc Med 154:11–15
32. Bergstrom M, Ericson K, Levander B et al (1977) Computed tomography of cranial subdural and epidural hematomas: variation of attenuation related to time and clinical events such as rebleeding. J Comput Assist Tomogr 1:449–455
33. Sargent S, Kennedy JG, Kaplan JA (1996) "Hyperacute" subdural hematoma: CT mimic of recurrent episodes of bleeding in the setting of child abuse. J Forensic Sci 41:314–316
34. Chen CY, Huang CC, Zimmerman RA et al (2001) High resolution cranial ultrasound in the shaken-baby syndrome. Neuroradiology 43:653–661
35. Vowles GH, Scholtz CL, Cameron JM (1987) Diffuse axonal injury in early infancy. J Clin Pathol 40:185–189
36. Kemp AM, Stoodley N, Cobley C et al (2003) Apnoea and brain swelling in non-accidental head injury. Arch Dis Child 88(6):472–476
37. Ewing-Cobbs L, Prasad M, Kramer L et al (2000) Acute neuroradiologic findings in young children with inflicted or noninflicted traumatic brain injury. Childs Nerv Syst 16:25–33
38. Feldman KW, Weinberger E, Milstein JM et al (1997) Cervical spine MRI in abused infants. Child Abuse Negl 21:199–205
39. Geddes JF, Vowles GH, Hackshaw AK et al (2001) Neuropathology of inflicted head injury in children. II Microscopic brain injury in infants. Brain 124:1299–1306
40. Conway EE Jr (1998) Nonaccidental head injury in infants: "the shaken baby syndrome revisited". Pediatr Ann 27:677–690
41. Nassogne MC, Sharrard M, Hertz-Pannier L et al (2002) Massive subdural haematomas in Menkes disease mimicking shaken baby syndrome. Childs Nerv Syst 18:729–731
42. Valentini D, Barbuti D, Grandin A et al (2011) A good growth in a child with scurvy. BMJ Case Reports
43. Paterson CR (2009) Temporary brittle bone disease: fractures in medical care. Acta Paediatr 98:1935–1938

Informed Consent and Medicolegal Issues Related to the Imaging of Pediatric Traumatic Emergencies

8

Antonio Pinto and Luigia Romano

8.1 Introduction

Informed consent represents a communication method that is ethically required before the beginning of any procedure or treatment [1]. It provides significant information concerning the diagnosis and the treatment of a patient. Consent is considered "valid" or "real" when it is given voluntary without any act of coercion by a person with capacity and competence to provide the consent; moreover, consent should include a minimum level of adequate information in relation to the nature of procedure to which he/she is consenting [2].

The legal implications and ethics of consent related to practice involving children are complex, especially in the emergency department (ED).

Minors (persons under the age of legal consent as defined by state law) frequently require care in the prehospital environment and present to the ED with nonsurgical or surgical conditions. Children occasionally present to the ED unaccompanied by a parent or legal guardian. Health-care professionals should desist from providing nonurgent testing and treatment to children who present to medical facilities unaccompanied by a custodial parent or legal guardian. If an emergency medical condition exists, the performance of the medical screening examinations and the stabilization of the pediatric patient must not be delayed.

A. Pinto (✉) • L. Romano
Department of Diagnostic Radiological Imaging, A. Cardarelli Hospital,
Via Cardarelli 9, Naples I-80131, Italy
e-mail: antopin1968@libero.it; luigia.romano@fastwebnet.it

V. Miele, M. Trinci (eds.), *Imaging Trauma and Polytrauma in Pediatric Patients*,
DOI 10.1007/978-3-319-08524-1_8

8.2 Informed Consent in the Pediatric Patient

If a parent or legal guardian is present or available, the health-care professional treating the child should make every reasonable effort to obtain and document informed consent [3].

If an emergency medical condition exists, including life- or limb-threatening conditions, severe pain, and surgical or nonsurgical conditions with the potential for severe harm or dysfunction if left untreated, the performance of the medical screening examinations and the stabilization of the pediatric patient, with an identified emergency medical condition, must not be delayed. Medical screening examination might require the use of extensive ED resources, including laboratory testing, diagnostic imaging, and subspecialty consultations, as needed for a correct diagnosis. The ethical basis for this approach is based in the professional's duty to search for the best interest of the child. The legal basis for taking action in an emergency when consent is not available is known as the "emergency exception rule" [3].

Under the emergency exception rule, a medical professional may presume consent and proceed with correct treatment and transport if the following four conditions are met:

1. The child is suffering from an emergent medical or surgical condition that places his or her life or health in danger.
2. The child's legal guardian is absent, unavailable, or unable to provide consent for treatment or transport.
3. Treatment or transport cannot be safely delayed until consent can be obtained.
4. The professional administers only treatment for emergent conditions [3].

The emergency exception exists to protect the health-care professional from liability with the postulation that if the parents were present, they would consent to the treatment [4].

If radiologic procedures are nonemergent, final responsibility for ensuring informed consent rests with the radiologist. The radiologist is the one performing and interpreting the examination and being compensated for doing so [5]. The radiologist usually has the best understanding of the proposed procedure and other imaging alternatives.

The essential components of consent includes voluntariness (willingness of patient to undergo treatment), capacity (patient is able to understand the nature of the treatment), and knowledge (adequate information about the nature of treatment are disclosed to the patient) [2]. Basic elements related to the content of the informed consent form that may be addressed before beginning of any treatment or procedure are the following: nature and need of procedure, risks, benefits, alternatives, and consequences of refusal of treatment.

In general, informed consent discussions should take place in quiet and private places. Patients who find themselves in an unfamiliar environment, preoccupied by pain or discomfort, and anxious over their condition often experience added difficulty in concentrating on what a physician or a radiologist is saying [6].

A particularly challenging condition occurs when the health-care professional is faced with a legal guardian who refuses to give consent for treatment of a child in situations in which such treatment is considered indispensable to the child's well-being. When a legal guardian refuses to consent to medical care or transport that is necessary and likely to prevent death, disability, or serious harm to the child, it might be necessary to notify the police and enlist their assistance in placing the child in temporary protective custody. In a life-threatening emergency, it might be necessary to involve hospital security so that emergent evaluation and treatment can begin while child-protective services and the police are notified [3].

If a language obstacle exists, informed consent for medical treatment should, when clinical circumstances permit, be obtained through a trained medical interpreter. Using an interpreter not only increases the likelihood of truly informed consent but also enhances the possibility of optimal medical treatment by allowing the professional to obtain accurate information about the child's underlying medical conditions, allergies, current medications, or other relevant and essential information.

Health care of older children and adolescents is complex as they are in the phase of developing competence to take part in decision making on their health. A child's agreement to medical procedures in situations where he or she is not legally authorized or lacks sufficient understanding for giving consent competently is called "assent." Children are considered to be "assent" when they have sufficient competence to understand the nature, risks, and benefits of a procedure, but not enough competence to give fully informed consent [7].

8.3 Medicolegal Issues

Injuries are one of the leading causes of mortality and morbidity among children in the United States [8]. As a result, evaluation of the current trend in the use of computed tomography (CT) for hospitalized pediatric trauma patients is of crucial importance from both potential health risk and financial perspectives.

Moreover, the pediatric population may be more sensitive than the adult population to the effects of ionizing radiation associated with medical imaging and in particular CT [9, 10].

The use of medical imaging techniques, including those using ionizing radiation, has increased exponentially over the past decades. Due to the evolving knowledge of the potential carcinogenic effects associated with radiation, imaging procedures that do not deliver ionizing radiation, such as MRI and ultrasound, should be optimized and used whenever possible and also in emergency situations, in the pediatric population.

It is rational to do everything that the radiologists can to try to use only the necessary amount of radiation in performing imaging studies of children. Radiologists have the responsibility to adequately inform clinical colleagues and patients about the risks and benefits of radiologic examinations. Efforts should be directed toward improved information and communication.

In nonemergency medical conditions, requirement for informed consent for CT scanning in children would inevitably raise specific concerns. These concerns would include the rights of parents or legal caretakers to refuse consent for an appropriately indicated CT examination. In such an event, the medical team can listen to the concerns of parents and patients [11], explain the benefits of CT scanning, and outline strategies adopted by radiologists to reduce radiation dose in children compared with the strategies in adults [5].

8.4 Conclusions

As a general rule, health-care professionals should always do what they believe to be in the best interest of the minor.

References

1. Berkowitz KA, Foglia MB, Chanko BL (2004) Informed consent. Chest 125:2367–2368
2. Kaushik JS, Narang M, Agarwal N (2010) Informed consent in pediatric practice. Indian Pediatr 47:1039–1046
3. Committee on Pediatric Emergency Medicine and Committee on Bioethics (2011) Consent for emergency medical services for children and adolescents. Pediatrics 128:427–433
4. American Academy of Pediatrics, Committee on Bioethics (1995) Informed consent, parental permission, and assent in pediatric practice. Pediatrics 95:314–317
5. Karsli T, Kalra MK, Self JL et al (2009) What physicians think about the need for informed consent for communicating the risk of cancer from low-dose radiation. Pediatr Radiol 39:917–925
6. Gunderman RB, Kakarala B (2012) Informed consent in professionalism. AJR Am J Roentgenol 198:W415–W416
7. Foreman DM (1999) The family rule: a framework for obtaining ethical consent for medical interventions from children. J Med Ethics 25:491–496
8. Roudsari BS, Psoter KJ, Vavilala MS et al (2013) CT use in hospitalized pediatric trauma patients: 15-year trends in a level I pediatric and adult trauma center. Radiology 267:479–486
9. Brody AS, Frush DP, Huda W et al (2007) Radiation risk to children from computed tomography. Pediatrics 120:677–682
10. Brenner DJ, Hall EJ (2007) Computed tomography: an increasing source of radiation exposure. N Engl J Med 357:2277–2284
11. Larson DB, Rader SB, Forman HP et al (2007) Informing parents about CT radiation exposure in children: it's OK to tell them. AJR Am J Roentgenol 189:271–275

MIX
Papier aus verantwortungsvollen Quellen
Paper from responsible sources
FSC® C105338

If you have any concerns about our products,
you can contact us on
ProductSafety@springernature.com

In case Publisher is established outside the EU,
the EU authorized representative is:
Springer Nature Customer Service Center GmbH
Europaplatz 3, 69115 Heidelberg, Germany

Printed by Libri Plureos GmbH
in Hamburg, Germany